Schizophrenia

A workbook for healthcare professionals

Edited by
Peter Thompson

Principal Lecturer
School of Health and Human Sciences
Liverpool John Moores University

RADCLIFFE MEDICAL PRESS

©2000 Liverpool John Moores University

Radcliffe Medical Press Ltd
18 Marcham Road, Abingdon, Oxon OX14 1AA

British Library Cataloguing in Publication Data

A catalogue record for this book is available from the British Library.

ISBN 1 85775 461 1

SMC

616.8982 THO

Typeset by Advance Typesetting Ltd, Oxon
Printed and bound by TJ International Ltd, Padstow, Cornwall

CONTENTS

STUDENT GUIDELINES – HOW TO USE THIS BOOK

This is intended as a self-study workbook, so you can choose when and where, and at what pace you study. The book is divided into chapters, each covering a particular aspect of the subject area. From time to time, as you read through the text, you will be asked to carry out tasks such as reflecting upon what you have read, thinking about the material in relation to your own experiences or expectations. These activities are designed for you to get as much out of the book as possible. They are important in helping you to consider and appraise the body of work being presented, particularly how it might apply to a primary care setting.

EXPLANATION OF ICONS

All chapters will invite you to participate in activities. These activities will take the following forms.

Writing and feedback

You may be asked to write down information – either in short list or descriptive form. This material may then be used to compare your opinions or knowledge base with that of the author who will give you some feedback within the context of the written material following the exercise. Such feedback may represent factual information or it may be representative of the author's opinion of those areas where you are asked for your personal observations.

Reading

The book cannot hope to address all of the relevant issues in any great depth. It is geared towards introducing concepts, informing about relevant theory and research, raising awareness and stimulating interest in finding out more. In this sense you will find the references quoted useful for further reading. You may find that some of the information will be useful in helping to form a resource for discussions or education sessions with patients, patients' families or colleagues.

Reflection

You will be asked to reflect upon the material presented, or on a question raised, and relate it to either your personal lifestyle or to your professional practice. These exercises are crucial in helping you to relate theoretical aspects to practice.

KEY WORDS AND PHRASES

Certain key words or phrases will be emphasised in the text; usually these will be explained in more detail later, perhaps after you have had a chance to reflect upon possible meanings or implications.

Occasionally there will not be enough space to develop certain themes or avenues of enquiry. In these instances the words in bold will point to areas where you may wish to read further, providing the relevant search term.

SELF-ASSESSMENT

At the end of each chapter, you will be invited to complete a short self-assessment exercise. This will enable you to check your progress in relation to the material covered within the chapter. Answers are given at the back of the book.

It is important to realise that to become a skilled practitioner in the systematic implementation of psychosocial interventions requires intensive practical training and appropriate supervision. This book does not provide this, but will offer some pointers to where those interested might seek further training.

We hope you will enjoy working through this material and that the knowledge you acquire will help in the delivery of services in your practice.

LIST OF CONTRIBUTORS

Mick McKeown is a lecturer/practitioner in mental health nursing, teaching at the University of Liverpool and working in clinical practice and staff development at North Mersey Community NHS Trust.

Ged McCann is County Development Officer for establishment and provision of inter-agency services for mentally disordered offenders in Yorkshire, and a lecturer in psychosocial interventions at the University of York.

Bob Cooper is Clinical Facilitator for adult mental health (community) services for North Mersey Community NHS Trust.

CHAPTER 1
An introduction to psychosocial interventions

This distance-learning pack provides an introduction to the concept of psychosocial interventions in the care of schizophrenia in primary care settings. It appears at an interesting time in the history of provision of services for this client group. The last decade has witnessed the arrival at an important juncture in the shift towards community care, with the last of the large mental hospital retraction programmes winding down. This trend began in the 1950s with a more enlightened post-war approach to social policy, notably a rejection of the institutionalising effects of the Victorian asylum system, and the advent of the first effective physical treatment for schizophrenia, in neuroleptic medication.

Despite the progressive nature of this policy shift, the varying degrees of poverty of outcome for many of this client group can be seen to be at least partly due to a perceived clinical impotence on the part of service providers. Clinicians have felt largely powerless, despite the benefits of medication, to prevent deterioration in social functioning and quality of life for the majority of people diagnosed schizophrenic, or to predict or prevent the disabling cycle of relapse which for so many typifies the course of this disorder. This therapeutic pessimism was reflected in an observed drift by practitioners away from the care of people with long-term problems toward providing brief interventions for less severe mental conditions. However, the psychosocial approach provides an antidote to vexed claims that nothing seems to work. If we couple this with innovations in the pharmacological management of symptoms, with the development of new atypical neuroleptics which arguably improve both therapeutic effect and minimise side effects, then it would seem that we are in a position to abandon previous pessimism and, perhaps for the first time, embrace a new-found clinical optimism toward this needy group of service users.

Of course, the success or failure of community care policies are as much a function of politics, economics and social attitudes as the activity of community-based practitioners. There is a real need to improve the social welfare and status of the severely mentally ill who have consistently been stigmatised, discriminated against and marginalised in contemporary society. Tackling these issues will be as difficult a task as ensuring the provision of quality, evidence-based services. However, neither will be completely successful without the other.

WHAT ARE PSYCHOSOCIAL INTERVENTIONS?

In one sense, the term 'psychosocial intervention' can be applied to any form of therapeutic interaction which has psychological and social dimensions. For instance, you may be aware of psychosocial approaches to palliative care, which involve a dying person's family, or you may have heard of different forms of counselling referred to as psychosocial in nature.

For the purposes of this book we will be working with a much narrower definition of psychosocial interventions. We are concerned with psychosocial interventions used in the care of people with **severe and enduring** mental health problems, usually having a diagnosis of **schizophrenia**. In this context, a number of clinical approaches have been developed and researched, demonstrating effectiveness in the management of the **diversity of problems** such people may face. It is these interventions which are now, somewhat fashionably, called **psychosocial interventions**. The term is often abbreviated and you may see or hear psychosocial interventions referred to as **PSI**. We will make use of this abbreviation from this point on.

Based upon a particular understanding of the course and nature of **psychotic problems** which emphasises the importance of stress in people's lives, **PSI** are used to reduce stress and improve coping. They do so either by modifying the social environment in some way, or by enhancing people's coping strategies.

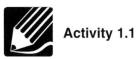 **Activity 1.1**

You may have used, or worked with people who have used, interventions which have been intended to reduce stress or improve coping. Think about these interventions and list them here.

Feedback to Activity 1.1

You may have identified a range of interventions which you consider to fit the description of PSI. They can be broadly categorised as follows:

- **anything that reduces stress or its impact** – either by modifying the social environment in some way, or by enhancing people's coping strategies. These interventions might include:

    - anxiety management sessions

    - taught relaxation techniques

    - distraction (like listening to music)

- **family therapy incorporating:**

    - psycho-education

    - communication skills training

    - problem-solving skills training

- **cognitive behavioural therapy** for psychotic symptoms

- **early warning signs monitoring.**

These are strategies and techniques which will be discussed in detail later in the book.

WHY PSYCHOSOCIAL INTERVENTIONS?

Government policy insists that mental health services prioritise the needs of people with the severest problems. This has led to the coining of the term '**severe and enduring mental illness**' to describe the target group. Apart from the observation that those in greatest need exert most demand on services, this focus can be seen to be at least partly motivated by concerns around the community management of vulnerability and risk. A number of high-profile incidents involving seriously mentally ill people have raised the anxieties of politicians, professionals and the general public.

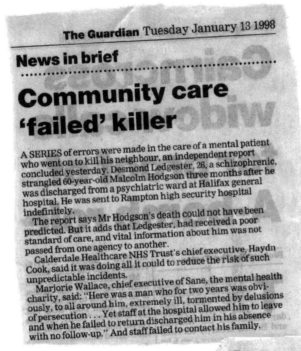

The Guardian Tuesday January 13 1998

News in brief

Community care 'failed' killer

A SERIES of errors were made in the care of a mental patient who went on to kill his neighbour, an independent report concluded yesterday. Desmond Ledgester, 26, a schizophrenic, strangled 60-year-old Malcolm Hodgson three months after he was discharged from a psychiatric ward at Halifax general hospital. He was sent to Rampton high security hospital indefinitely.

The report says Mr Hodgson's death could not have been predicted. But it adds that Ledgester, had received a poor standard of care, and vital information about him was not passed from one agency to another.

Calderdale Healthcare NHS Trust's chief executive, Haydn Cook, said it was doing all it could to reduce the risk of such unpredictable incidents.

Marjorie Wallace, chief executive of Sane, the mental health charity, said: "Here was a man who for two years was obviously, to all around him, extremely ill, tormented by delusions of persecution . . . Yet staff at the hospital allowed him to leave and when he failed to return discharged him in his absence with no follow-up." And staff failed to contact his family.

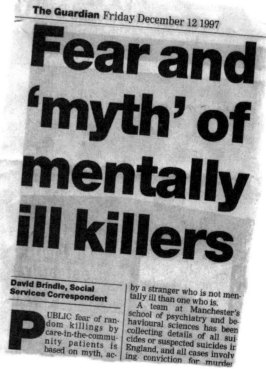

The Guardian Friday December 12 1997

Fear and 'myth' of mentally ill killers

David Brindle, Social Services Correspondent

PUBLIC fear of random killings by care-in-the-community patients is based on myth, ac-

by a stranger who is not mentally ill than one who is.

A team at Manchester's school of psychiatry and behavioural sciences has been collecting details of all suicides or suspected suicides in England, and all cases involving conviction for murder

---

Though the risk of this client group committing serious crimes such as murder or assault is an important concern, such incidents are relatively rare. It is probably more likely that people with severe mental health problems are vulnerable to harm and at risk themselves. The suicide rate in this group is many times greater than for others, and this is reflected in the national targets provided by successive government initiatives (DoH, 1993; 1998a).

There is a general and progressive policy trend towards a primary care-led NHS (DoH, 1996a) grounded in evidence-based practice, and this is to be welcomed. However, it must be realised that traditional models of preventive medicine and health promotion are not particularly appropriate to the long-term, continuing needs and problems presented by our stated client group and their carers. Yet, the accompanying policy goal of deinstitutionalisation has firmly placed the care of people with severe and enduring mental health problems in the community, defining a central role for practitioners in primary care. There are several good reasons for developing psychosocial therapies within this service context, not least the concentration of people within the community who would meet the definition of suffering a severe and enduring mental illness. There are large numbers not necessarily in regular contact with services and many are homeless. An examination of the current levels of service provision for this client group points to ways in which quality may be improved.

Both the Butterworth Report (Mental Health Nursing Review Team, 1994) and the Clinical Standards Advisory Group Report (1995) recommend that practitioners prioritise efforts on those with a severe and enduring mental illness, and that a wide range of psychosocial interventions ought to be offered to service users. These recommendations are expected to inform the forthcoming National Service Frameworks for mental health (DoH, 1998b). Staff will therefore need to be appropriately informed in the relevant knowledge base and trained in specific skills. Attempts to ensure the creation of seamless services across different care provision settings and agencies will flounder unless there is some sort of common conceptual framework or 'currency' informing a consistency of interventive strategies.

However, if we investigate the services available to this client group within community or hospital settings there is an absence of systematic psychosocial intervention. This has been the consistent finding of major reviews of community psychiatric nursing activity, National Clinical Standards (CSAG, 1995) and the recent Mental Health Act Commission/Sainsbury Centre (1997) scrutiny of in-patient services. For many patients it is not clear what treatments are available other than medication. Despite widespread use of neuroleptics, large numbers of patients continue to experience persistent symptoms. There is a lack of family involvement and relatives' needs are largely unmet. Consequently, many patients and relatives have a poor opinion and limited expectations of services.

Yet, a body of research which originates in the early days of community care with the commencement of the closure of the old Victorian asylums in the late 1950s suggests a basis for better quality services. Sound case management and the delivery of psychosocial interventions are the most effective means of maintaining this group in the community and ensuring optimal outcomes in a number of desirable areas. Indeed, psychosocial approaches used in the management of people with schizophrenia are amongst the few non-pharmacological therapies available which have been subject to rigorous scientific evaluation. All of this research points to vastly improved outcomes if psychosocial interventions are used in conjunction with effectively prescribed medication. It is these psychosocial interventions and the underpinning research which we will detail in this book, and explore the potential for their implementation in primary care settings like general practice. But before we do this we must attempt to define some terms, such as **severe and enduring mental illness, psychotic problems** and **schizophrenia**, and say something about what the experience of these conditions is like.

SEVERE AND ENDURING MENTAL HEALTH PROBLEMS

Despite the recognised need to coordinate services towards meeting the needs of the severely mentally ill, there is a lack of consensus in how this group is to be defined.

 Activity 1.2

You may or may not have heard of the term 'severe and enduring mental illness'. It is the term used to cover a range of long-term mental health problems. Consider the term now. What images come to mind about patients so described? What are the needs of such individuals?

Feedback to Activity 1.2

Within your practice you may have some experience of individuals with severe and enduring mental illness, and you may have some difficulty in defining their needs clearly. Broad guidance in relation to defining this group is given in the Health of the Nation policy document *Building Bridges: a guide to arrangements for inter-agency working for the care and protection of severely mentally ill people* (DoH, 1995). This booklet suggests that individuals suffering from severe mental illness can be identified as having some or all of the following features:

1 a diagnosis of a mental illness

2 substantial disability resulting from their illness, for example in terms of self-care, employment or relationships

3 currently have marked symptoms; or suffer from a chronic, enduring condition

4 have had several relapses or recurrent crises, leading to frequent contact with services

5 are seen to constitute a significant risk, either to their own safety or that of others.

In practice, the typical groups of diagnoses defined as belonging to this category include:

• psychotic illness

• dementia

• severe neurotic illness

• personality disorder

• developmental disorder (learning difficulties).

Leaving aside organic problems like dementia for the moment, the reality is that people with psychotic problems easily constitute the largest group within such definitions of severe mental illness; and of these, people who have been diagnosed as schizophrenic are the most numerous. Indeed, it is often the case that the term 'severe and enduring mental illness' is used interchangeably with the term 'schizophrenia', and you may have used this term in your response to Activity 1.2.

Though many of the interventions we will go on to describe and much of the research which underpins them, have relevance to wider groups, particularly in other forms of psychotic illness, it is the support and treatment of schizophrenia sufferers and their families with which we will concern ourselves in this book.

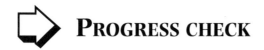 **PROGRESS CHECK**

In this chapter you have been introduced to the concept of psychosocial interventions used as an approach to caring for individuals suffering from mental health problems.

Before considering this in more depth you are now invited to check your progress and ensure that you understand the material covered so far. Please answer the following questions and check your answers with those given in Appendix 1.

1 What are psychosocial interventions (PSI)?

2 What client groups in particular may benefit from the use of PSI, and why?

3 List three examples of PSI.

If after checking your progress you are still unsure, then please refer back to the relevant part of the material within the chapter or undertake further reading as advised within.

When you are sure that you understand the material, move on to Chapter 2 which explores the nature of schizophrenia and explains why and how PSI are potentially beneficial to the individual sufferer and family.

CHAPTER 2
Understanding the client group and family needs

Section 1 – The nature of schizophrenia

Within this section we shall be defining and exploring schizophrenia. We will build up a picture of the characteristics of schizophrenia and determine the treatment options, both medical and psychological, which are available.

This material may be new to you, or it may provide you with an opportunity to review your understanding of this group of problems. Either way, the chapter should prove useful to you in ensuring that you identify those areas of patient need which may be the focus of using PSI.

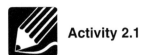 **Activity 2.1**

Before going on to consider schizophrenia in more detail, it may be useful to establish some details about your caseload. Take a few minutes to consider patients within your practice and answer the following questions:

1 How many patients in total?

2 How many of these (number and/or percentage) have a diagnosis of schizophrenia?

3 Make a list of the problems you associate with the diagnosis of schizophrenia.

You may have identified few or many patients within your caseload who have a diagnosis of schizophrenia, and you will realise that this diagnosis is given to people who may suffer from a range of distressing problems and symptoms. These problems can affect all aspects of a person's life – their thoughts, feelings and actions.

People can have all sorts of strange experiences such as hearing voices, seeing things, having mixed-up thoughts, feeling that they are being controlled or that other people are going to harm them, and a lack of drive or energy to do things. These problems are often called '**psychotic**' symptoms. The psychotic symptoms are usually divided into the categories of '**positive**' and '**negative**' symptoms. The positive symptoms include **hallucinations**, **delusions** and **thought disorder**, these being phenomena that are 'added in' to a person's range of experiences. The negative symptoms are all those things that are seemingly 'taken away' from people, such as the ability to action certain behaviours, e.g. getting out of bed, getting dressed, washing etc.

Anxiety and **depression** are also common in people with schizophrenia. It is often the case that schizophrenia sufferers also have a range of **social problems**. They can become poverty stricken, unemployed or homeless. Their relationships can become fraught, or break down altogether, leading to a degree of social isolation. Importantly, people with a diagnosis of schizophrenia are at a greater risk of **suicide**.

Not everybody will have all the symptoms, nor be affected in completely the same way. The problems of schizophrenia usually occur in 'attacks' or episodes. Some people may only have a first episode, never having another. Others will have repeated episodes called **relapses**, being relatively well in between. Even those who have some degree of recovery might still have some symptoms which persist. Professional staff and family and friends have an important role in helping people stay as well as possible.

There are many myths about schizophrenia. Some people think it is a 'split personality' or that sufferers are likely to be unusually violent. Both of these things are not true.

Schizophrenia is not rare. People have a lifetime risk of one chance in a hundred of being affected. Though nobody really knows what causes schizophrenia, it is thought that **stress** is very important. A good way of understanding what happens is to think of people as being born with a **vulnerability** of developing the problems of schizophrenia when faced with certain levels of stress. If the level of stress is greater than a person's vulnerability threshold, then it is at these times that people will show symptoms. This is not to say that stress causes schizophrenia, but it does mean that stress will bring on episodes, or make symptoms worse. People may be affected by the stress of major life events such as bereavements or divorce, or ongoing things such as tension or arguments at home or work.

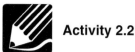 **Activity 2.2**

Looking back to the patients identified in Activity 2.1, think about what you offer as a caring professional. For example, you may be involved in other interventions such as facilitating support groups or organising educational input.

Feedback to Activity 2.2

The usual treatment is long-term **medication**, taken even when symptoms are under control. Other important sources of help are those therapies described as psychosocial interventions which we describe in this book. These involve working with sufferers and other important people such as family, friends or carers in an attempt, together, to reduce the impact of stress in people's lives.

DIAGNOSING SCHIZOPHRENIA

If we think of diagnosis as the process by which doctors review people's symptoms and problems and then say what illness a person is suffering from, then this can usually be a lot more straightforward in general medicine than in psychiatry. This is partly because of the fact that it is much easier to understand a person's physical problems in terms of illnesses with obvious symptoms, clearly defined causes and possible medical cures.

The sorts of problems that people seek help for from psychiatry and mental health services are often complex, and not easily understood or dealt with in simple terms. It is also the nature of some mental health problems to make it difficult for people to tell their doctor exactly *what* the problem seems to be. Or people may be reluctant to talk about their problems because of emotional distress or feelings of suspicion, guilt or embarrassment. It helps a lot if people are as cooperative as they are able to be.

A psychiatrist will look for certain symptoms, usually of mental state, and hope to be able to diagnose the person as suffering from a particular psychiatric disease category. This is made harder again by the fact that certain of the more common symptoms of mental distress – anxiety and depression for instance – are found in more than one psychiatric illness. So the assessment may be looking for clusters or collections of symptoms. Assessment will involve interviewing the person and their family and friends, looking for additional information relating to family history, behaviours normal to the patient and details of any changes from the established norm for that individual. It may also be necessary to observe *and* talk to people over time, perhaps in a hospital ward, to be able to make an appropriate diagnosis.

POTENTIAL STIGMA

Unfortunately, for many people, merely being described as having a mental illness or mental health problem can result in damaging consequences. Other people may react to the labelled person negatively as a result of stigma. For all of these reasons a psychiatrist may sometimes be reluctant to attach a diagnostic label *too* quickly.

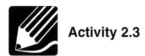 **Activity 2.3**

Reflect upon this reluctance to attach a label too quickly and try to identify advantages and disadvantages of doing so.

Advantages   **Disadvantages**

 Feedback to Activity 2.3

Advantages	Disadvantages
Allows timely and effective commencement of treatment, thus relieving symptoms.	Stigma and being shunned by family and friends.
Helps family to understand and play an active role in treatment.	Reactive depression and anxiety.

However, a balance has to be struck because some types of disorder, including schizophrenia, might be particularly amenable to *early* intervention.

Some people may reject their diagnosis, perhaps because they do not realise they have a problem or they fear the stigma of being a mental patient. Other people are only too glad to accept a diagnosis because this can provide an explanation for previously inexplicable experiences or actions. Whatever the given diagnosis, it is important to remember that this need not be cast in stone, and may change as more information about a person's problems comes to light. Regardless of diagnosis, or feelings about it, healthcare staff need to attempt to work with the symptoms people complain of. A **problem-centred approach** to working with patients is most appropriate for utilising psychosocial interventions; however, we must be aware that the problems schizophrenia sufferers are likely to want help with are more likely to be complicated than simple.

COMPLEXITY OF PROBLEMS

No two schizophrenia sufferers will have exactly the same set of problems. Even if they have similar problems, they may be interlinked with different problems, or have different causative factors. This can be illustrated by thinking about just one problem which is relatively common among people with a schizophrenia diagnosis. Such people can become socially isolated, even to the extent of staying in their bed for long periods during the day. For one person this may be due to the fact that they experience distressing voices, which get worse when they are around other people, so staying in bed is an attempt to manage the social environment to minimise hallucinatory experiences. For others, this staying in bed might be because of a diminished ability to initiate the act of getting out of bed – a negative symptom. If a person is depressed, perhaps with associated low self-esteem, then they may feel physically and emotionally drained of energy to the extent that they find it hard to get out of bed, or difficult to face people. If anxiety is a problem this might get worse in particular situations such as going out of the house, and might be minimised by retreating from social contact. Similarly, worrying thoughts or delusional ideas like paranoia can make people fearful and withdrawn. Depression, anxiety, hearing voices, or frightening thoughts and beliefs can all result in disturbed sleep patterns, which might result in people having to sleep during the day or feeling too tired to get out of bed. Neuroleptic medication can have a marked sedative effect, leaving people over-tired and drained of energy. Conversely, because a long-term feature of schizophrenia can be a disintegration of social networks and deterioration of ordinary patterns of activity, people's lives can become empty to the extent that they feel they have little that is pleasurable to do during the day and thus lack any worthwhile incentive to get out of bed.

Another important but often overlooked issue is the effect of other people's reactions to people with schizophrenia. It may be the case that a person either looks or behaves a little or even very oddly in public. They may face a variety of reactions, including ridicule, fearful withdrawal or even outright hostility. This may be evidenced by the overt and obvious behaviour of others, or more subtly by facial expressions, dismissive glances or whispered comments. Such responses do not necessarily need the trigger of strange appearance or bizarre behaviour, and can be expressed merely in the knowledge that a person, perhaps a neighbour, carries the schizophrenia label. The net effect of such stigma can result in a form of discrimination where people who are seen as different in this respect are effectively excluded from ordinary social interactions, or begin to exclude themselves because of the reactions of other people.

Just by contemplating what might, on the surface, have seemed the relatively simple and easily understood problem of spending too much time in bed, we can conclude that it is likely to be much more complex. Any person with this problem may find that in their case it has a number of contributory features, and it is difficult to help provide solutions unless we understand the complexity of how these might interact. Figure 2.1 shows one way in which we might divide up the sort of problems people with schizophrenia may experience. In a similar way to the problem discussed above, we can regard such groupings of symptoms or problems as an artificial device which may help in terms of pointing to areas which require systematic assessment, but can hide complex interactions between problems. It is important to remember this when planning care and support for individuals and their carers.

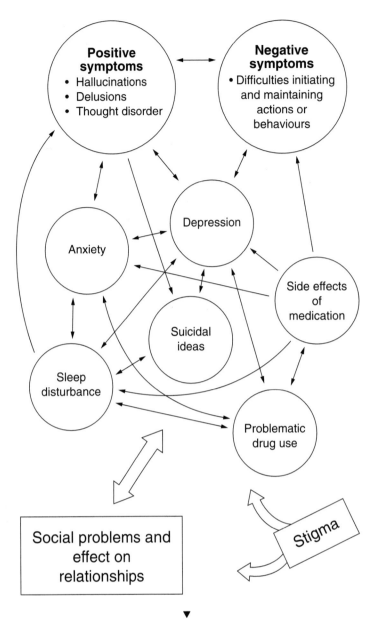

Figure 2.1 Groupings of problems (individuals may experience a combination of these – some may not be present).

In summarising Figure 2.1, the more common problems associated with schizophrenia are:

- hallucinations

- delusions

- thought disorder

- negative symptoms

- depression

- anxiety

- suicidal ideas

- problematic drug use

- sleep disturbance

- effects on relationships

- sexual problems

- stigma.

We will now consider these problems, and their impact on the individual and family, in more detail.

HALLUCINATIONS

People with psychosis can experience a range of altered perceptions which may become heightened or blunted. For example, a person might see colours either brighter or duller than normal. An **illusion** occurs when a person misperceives an actual object or event in their environment, e.g. seeing a cracked window pane as a spider's web. The most extreme form of disturbed perceptual experiences is hallucination, or perceiving something which is not actually there. Hallucinations can occur in any of the sensory domains (visual, olfactory, gustatory, tactile or auditory), but the most common are **auditory hallucinations**, usually in the form of hearing voices.

Hearing voices

If a person hears a voice or voices when there is no explanation at all for the source then this is an example of an auditory hallucination. Such voices can sound as if they come from the room or from some object or from another part of the body, but there will be nobody there who can be seen to be talking. The voices will be heard as if through the ears, like any other sound with a more obvious source. Sometimes people get voices but think that they are heard as if in the mind or inside the head. These are called **pseudo auditory hallucinations**.

 Activity 2.4

Try to imagine hearing a voice, or perhaps some music. You look around but cannot locate its source. To make matters worse the voice mentions your name. How do you think you would feel and react?

Many people have had the experience of hearing voices, and this is not always due to a mental illness. Even people who have a psychiatric diagnosis can prefer to think of their voices in non-medical terms. However, to experience hallucinations for no apparent reason usually results in the diagnosis of some form of psychotic mental health problem. Indeed, it is the often distressing consequences of hearing voices which can lead people or their families to seek help from services. The voices can be very loud, they can say upsetting things, or can command people to do things that they would not ordinarily do. Sometimes the voice might be just a whisper or muttering and it is difficult to make out any words. Or people might hear other sounds like tapping or music. There could be one voice, or many different voices. The voices might come and go in any day, or from day to day, or from week to week. They might be there all the time, but more intense at different times of the day. Not all voices are unpleasant – some people might enjoy experiencing their voices, others might have a mixture of pleasant and unpleasant voices.

Particularly if the voices are very frequent, loud or critical they can cause a lot of disruption to people's lives. For instance it can become incredibly hard to concentrate or talk to other people if your thoughts are interrupted by voices. Also, if a voice is continually telling someone to do a thing, however strange or risky it might be, then it can be very hard to resist. Because voices can seem to speak directly to a person it is not uncommon for voice hearers to carry on conversations with their voices. This can cause embarrassment in public.

DELUSIONS

A common feature of schizophrenia is that people can hold beliefs which most other people would find strange or difficult to understand. Such irrational and seemingly unshakeable beliefs are called delusions.

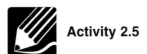 **Activity 2.5**

Imagine that you have been interviewed for a job. You were unsuccessful but were not given any explanation. How would you feel? What might you attribute your failure to?

 Feedback to Activity 2.5

We all have belief systems and respond to situations in relation to these. Usually the beliefs are reasonable and rational. For example, we may believe that the interviewers had already selected someone and that the interviews were just a question of going through the motions. However, if you believe that the interview panel were out to get you and that their denial of the job was part of some personal conspiracy, then you might have a problem.

Examples of delusional beliefs

Delusional beliefs can take many forms but some examples include:

- a person believing that everyone is against them or out to do them harm (this sort of delusion is called **paranoia** or paranoid ideas)

- a person believing that they are a very important person or that they have special powers (**grandiose** delusions)

- a person believing that items of news on the television or in the papers have special meaning for them (**ideas of reference**)

- a person believing that their thoughts are being spoken out loud in a way that other people can hear them (**thought broadcast**)

- a person believing that they are under the control of another person or an alien power (**ideas of passivity**)

- a person believing that their thoughts can be read by others, or that they can read other people's minds.

It may not be obvious that somebody has deluded beliefs if they do not talk about them. Some people may only contemplate their beliefs from time to time. However, others will readily discuss their delusional ideas if asked what they think, or can be so preoccupied by them that they dominate their thoughts. When this happens it can severely disrupt their life and relationships. People can begin to lose touch with reality altogether, and may call attention to themselves by saying and doing unusual things. Friends and family might react to this by either avoiding talking about the delusions or telling the person that they are wrong to believe such things. It is always best to take somebody's beliefs seriously and to listen when people want to talk about them.

A person with delusions may be completely convinced that what they believe is real (just as in the case of your assumptions about the reasons for not being given the job), even if this causes its own problems. However, it is not correct to assume that all delusions are held with absolute conviction. People might have doubts about their own beliefs, and this level of doubt might change with time or depending on circumstances. Because everybody uses their attitudes and beliefs to help them interpret what happens in their lives, delusions can lead to people misinterpreting events – a bit like the Everton or Liverpool fan who can see *no* good at all in the other side! In time, people gather a body of 'evidence' from the things which happen to them which they use to confirm what they believe. For example, a person who thinks that people can read his mind might look for people's facial expressions, like smiles or winks, which become the 'proof' that they are aware of what he is thinking at that time. Of course these other people will be smiling or winking for a completely different reason.

THOUGHT DISORDER

Thought disorder is a term applied to a number of problems which affect people's ability to communicate in an understandable way. The problems of thought disorder are examples of positive symptoms of psychosis. Even though they are called *thought* disorder, they are recognised because of the effect on a person's speech. For this reason you might hear thought disorders referred to as **speech disorders**. Very few people suffer from severe and lasting speech problems. These usually resolve as people get generally better. However, attempts to understand and listen to people who have thought disorder are important. A person's communication can be improved and they will really appreciate those who make an effort to listen and help.

For some people their speech remains almost intact so that it can seem that it *should* make sense – the person speaks in sentences with more or less adequate punctuation. However, what they actually say can be completely irrelevant or make no sense. For others, the speech breaks down so much that it can seem just like a jumble of unconnected words. Sometimes words are used against their usual meaning, but manage to convey a particular meaning for that person, like in a metaphor. When this happens it can offer an insight into how that person is feeling, despite their difficulty in expressing themself (Kraepelin, cited in Kingdon *et al.*, 1994).

Examples of how these problems affect a person's ability to communicate include:

- rapid speech or pressure of speech – the speech is too quick to make sense of, words run into one another, there may be addition of unnecessary words

- very slow speech, or too long pauses, or no speech at all

- flight of ideas – shifts in topic occur with the speech progressing via odd links, like rhyming or punning

- speech may jump between ideas with no obvious link

- word salad – incoherent strings of unrelated words

- neologisms – the use of totally new words

- use of ordinary words or phrases in unusual ways

- irrelevant speech to the subject under discussion.

It can be upsetting and frustrating not to be able to get across to people what you mean. Perhaps you have experienced this within your work. From the patient's perspective, they may not realise just how difficult it is for others to understand them.

NEGATIVE SYMPTOMS

A feature of severe mental health problems can be a collection of symptoms which involve reduced drive, apathy and motivational difficulties. These are called 'negative symptoms'. They are called this because it appears that aspects of a person's usual behaviour are seemingly taken away. This is in contrast with 'positive symptoms', such as hearing voices, so-called because they are seemingly added in to people's experiences.

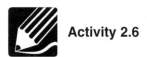 **Activity 2.6**

Make a list of your normal daily routine from rising in the morning to going to bed.

 Feedback to Activity 2.6

In your list you will probably have mentioned many routine daily activities which we take for granted. With schizophrenia, very often the person is unable or has diminished capacity to carry out these activities because of losing drive, interest and motivation. Possible negative symptoms include:

- withdrawal and avoidance of other people

- loss of energy

- taking longer to do things

- staying in bed

- not washing or looking after dress or appearance

- losing interest in things or people

- not doing a fair share of jobs around the house

- seeming loss of emotions or the expression of feelings

- expressing the 'wrong' feeling, such as laughing when talking about a serious issue.

Psychologists explain these symptoms in terms of problems *initiating* or *regulating* behaviours or actions. The person may have great difficulty starting off certain behaviours such as talking or getting up out of bed, or have difficulty controlling certain behaviours, resulting in, for instance, incongruous expression of feelings. It is very important to make this clear because sometimes people with negative symptoms can seem to be lazy or disinterested, and indeed are often described as such. This is not the case but such a view can cause arguments or stress at home. Because stress makes these symptoms worse, a vicious circle can develop if people are nagged or told to 'pull themselves together'. The best way of helping is to offer gentle encouragement, and to be clear and unambiguous about what is wanted in any request.

Although medication seems to help the positive symptoms there is no clear evidence that most neuroleptic medication helps the negative symptoms, although it is claimed that certain of the new **atypical neuroleptics** have such an effect. Unfortunately, because most of this medication has a sedative effect, negative symptoms can appear to become worse. If there is also accompanying depression, which is not uncommon, then it can be really difficult to work out what is causing a person's motivational problems.

DEPRESSION

Depressive features are commonly found in 25 to 40 per cent of people diagnosed as schizophrenic. There are varying degrees of low mood but when people are referred to as depressed, or diagnosed as clinically depressed, this means much more than just feeling sad or going through a bad patch. The major mental health problem of depression involves people feeling bad about almost every aspect of themselves or their lives. People who feel like this can experience a range of symptoms. These include inability to sleep, loss of appetite and weight loss, and seemingly overwhelming feelings of hopelessness, worthlessness and despair, accompanied with tearfulness or even uncontrollable weeping. They may feel guilty for no apparent or justifiable reason, or that they have lost the ability to feel. There may be a loss of drive, making even the simplest task seem difficult. When people experience such a low mood they might feel that they have no control at all over these symptoms, to the point where they cannot turn their attention to other things. There is a real risk of suicide when people are depressed. Some people with schizophrenia may not be able to explain why they feel depressed, for others their low mood may be related to pessimistic or hopeless thoughts about the future course of their illness, their quality of life, or in response to others' treatment and approaches towards them.

Anxiety is often also a feature of depressed people's problems, giving people repetitive and disturbing thoughts which turn over and over in their minds. In this state depressed people can feel incredibly tense and agitated, or threatened by things they cannot explain.

ANXIETY

Anxiety is a normal human emotion which everyone will feel at some time or other. This is an intense feeling of worry which can last for varying amounts of time and differ in severity. The effects of anxiety are not always negative – being a little nervous often helps us to perform well, say in a sporting event or when taking an exam. However, people with psychotic problems can suffer a range of different degrees of anxiety associated with their other symptoms.

Feelings of anxiety result from chemical changes in our body as it responds to a sense of 'threat'. This is often called the 'fight or flight' response. Hormones, such as adrenalin cause effects in the body such as a faster heartbeat, increased sweating, rapid breathing and tensing of muscles. All of these things make us ready to deal with whatever threatens us. However, problems which trigger anxiety in people nowadays are not the sort you might wish to, or be able to, fight or run away from. This can lead to feelings of anxiety staying with us for long periods. We also have uncomfortable feelings of anxiety when remembering things that make us anxious or thinking ahead to having to face such things. Such anxiety-provoking circumstances, the seemingly inescapable and worrying ruminations of precontemplation, can be a feature of psychotic illness. A degree of insight can lead to more general worries about what the future might hold.

When people are anxious for more than just fleeting periods they can experience a number of distressing problems. They may have headaches and muscle pain, butterflies in the stomach or even vomiting, dry mouth, loss of appetite, disturbed sleep, dizziness, bowel problems, anxious thoughts going round and round in the mind, and generally feel tired or exhausted. Anxiety feeds off itself in a vicious circle, with anxious thoughts leading on to greater levels of anxiety. When this happens very rapidly it is called a panic attack. People who have panic attacks may experience severe symptoms of anxiety together with thoughts that something absolutely awful is about to happen, or that they are out of control.

If people have severe anxiety or panic attacks associated with fear of particular things or situations, this may be referred to as a phobia. People may also become anxious about tasks such as washing their hands, to the extent that they feel compelled to repeatedly carry it out. If this happens to an extent where it severely disrupts a person's life, it is called an obsession or an obsessional-compulsive disorder.

SUICIDAL IDEAS

Suicide is a major cause of death in this country. People with a schizophrenia diagnosis have a tenfold greater risk than the general population. This might be due to the effects of severe depression, perhaps associated with insight and hopelessness, or people may commit irrational acts of self-harm as a consequence of commands made by voices, or be rendered vulnerable by specific delusional beliefs. It is difficult to imagine what somebody who contemplates such an act must be going through. Not everyone who thinks about suicide or attempts it will actually succeed in ending their life, but the aftermath of a person taking their own life devastates close family and friends.

Suicide is most common amongst young men. Overall it accounts for about one in every hundred of all deaths, but it is *preventable*. Professional staff, family and friends can all help to support and look after a person who feels like committing suicide. It can be helpful to have your problems listened to and engaged with by others. People in this position often have unbearable feelings of helplessness and hopelessness. They can be helped to gain hope and think about other ways of taking control of their lives. It is important that people who need such help are taken *seriously*. Often the degree to which a person is at risk can be weighed up on the basis of what they say. People might need to be questioned about their thoughts before they will talk about them. Remember, *talking about suicidal ideas can help*. Doing this sensitively will not plant the idea of committing suicide in people's minds, nor increase the risk of them acting upon such thoughts.

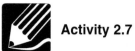 **Activity 2.7**

Think about patients within your caseload or practice population. What do you regard as being indications of serious suicidal intent? List them here.

Feedback to Activity 2.7

There are some general risk factors, but remember that they will not apply to every person. High-risk groups include:

- people who say they currently want to kill themselves

- people who have made a specific plan of how to do this

- people who have made active preparations, like buying tablets

- people who have already made suicide attempts – the risk increases if the previous attempts were recent (in the last month), or if the means chosen was felt by the person to have had a good chance of being lethal

- people who are depressed, or recovering from a depressive episode

- people who are actively psychotic, particularly if they hear voices telling them to harm themselves

- people with problems of drug use, including alcohol

- people who have experienced a significant bereavement.

If a person is thinking about suicide, or if somebody is worried about a person they know, they must be encouraged to *seek the help of others*.

PROBLEMATIC DRUG USE

It is becoming increasingly recognised that large numbers of people with severe and enduring mental health problems also have problems with drug use, most commonly alcohol but also including other drugs. This has led to the coining of the term '**dual diagnosis**' to describe people who have both sets of problems. People who have mental health problems probably use as many different drugs, legal or illegal, as anybody else. Some will find that they can do this without it having a worsening effect upon their mental well being. However, for others there may be an adverse effect upon their problems and symptoms, or the drug use might trigger off a relapse of their illness. It is important then that people with mental health problems give some serious thought to whatever drugs they take, and the effects that these might have. It is probably realistic to assume that, whether we may think certain drug use is harmful or not, people are unlikely to immediately stop using drugs on the say so of concerned professionals or family members. If people wish to continue taking certain drugs then they ought to be helped to take steps to do this as *safely* as possible. This sort of strategy is known as **harm reduction** or **harm minimisation**.

Just thinking in terms of the effects of drugs on people's mental or general health, sometimes the distinction between legal and illegal drugs is not particularly helpful. For instance, many people think that because certain drugs such as alcohol or nicotine (in tobacco) are legal, they are less harmful than illegal drugs such as heroin or cannabis. However, more people die every year from alcohol or smoking-related causes than for all other drugs put together. Most people think that the caffeine found in tea and coffee is quite harmless. But these stimulant drugs, and tobacco, which has the same effect, can make a lot of problems worse for people who have anxiety or psychosis. This is particularly the case if people drink or smoke heavily.

The reasons why people with mental health problems use drugs are likely to be similar, if not identical, to those expressed by the general public at large. The most obvious reason people use drugs is for pleasure. Other reasons include coping with stress, as a 'pick me up', blotting out pain or distress, helping to mix in company, improving self-esteem, going along with other people, to improve concentration or artistry, out of habit, or because it is difficult to stop. Some of these reasons might apply with more intensity to people with long-standing mental health problems, or they might have some reasons for using drugs which are quite specifically a result of their mental problems or how other people relate to them. These might include using drugs to 'self-medicate' symptoms (e.g. dampening down voices) or ameliorate the side effects of prescribed medication. Conversely, drug use can engender a degree of social interaction otherwise denied to people feeling lonely and isolated.

People who self-medicate might find that they can make one symptom better, but another gets worse; or they might be prepared to put up with a worsening of symptoms if the drug use has other positive effects, like opening up friendships. People with severe mental health problems might be more vulnerable to some of the negative effects of getting involved in illicit activity around drugs, and might get taken advantage of, or take more risks than they need to. Because some of this activity is illegal, it can be difficult for people who are involved to discuss any problems they might be having. Concerned practitioners, perhaps in liaison with the local drug treatment services, may be able to discuss options with people who have schizophrenia and use drugs problematically, and help plan what to do. They will not be in a position to make decisions for people, but will offer helpful advice and information.

SLEEP DISTURBANCE

People who suffer from a range of mental health or emotional problems often find that they have difficulties with their sleep. This is especially the case for schizophrenia sufferers. People who are depressed or anxious may find it difficult to get off to sleep at night, or find themselves waking much earlier than they wish to. People who hear voices or who have frightening thoughts can also find their sleep disturbed by these problems. It may be the case that these problems are themselves made worse by a lack of sleep. It is not uncommon for people who are emotionally disturbed or psychotic to have nightmares. An increase in dreaming can be a side effect of certain medication. Other drugs, like those in coffee, tea and cigarettes, or certain street drugs, have an energising effect on the body. This type of stimulation makes sleep problems worse.

Sometimes, when getting to sleep and staying asleep is very difficult it can seem that the whole night passes with no sleep at all. Usually this is not the case, and even when people are convinced this has happened they may have managed to get some sleep. One effect of neuroleptic or other medication is to make people drowsy and tired. Unfortunately this tiredness

---

does not always come on most strongly at night. This can lead to people being very sleepy during the day, whilst struggling to get to sleep when they want to. Similarly, some of the symptoms of depression or the negative symptoms of psychosis can lead people to be lethargic during the day, perhaps disrupting their sleeping pattern.

Sleep is a normal activity, and something that everyone must have to some extent to feel alert and refreshed. When we sleep our body repairs itself from the physical and emotional wears and tears of the day. Lack of sleep causes people to become irritable and to have difficulty thinking clearly. Because some people with severe mental health problems might be less active during the day, they might 'cat nap' from time to time. This snatching of little pockets of sleep can reduce the amount of sleep the body demands in the night, leading to night-time restlessness. Some people drink alcohol to help them sleep, but this will not help in the long term. The alcohol might help to induce sleep but its effects can also make people have to get up in the night.

The most important thing people with sleep problems can do to help themselves is to try hard to maintain a 'normal' sleep pattern. That is, sleeping at night rather than during the day, despite feeling very tired. This also means trying hard to wake at the same time each day. This is very difficult for people who have marked negative symptoms or are on a lot of medication. These things need to be discussed with the care team, who might be able to help. For instance, the timing or the dosage of medication might be changed so it has less impact on a person's sleeping pattern. People at home might be helped with encouragement to keep active during the day so that they get their sleep at night.

Cutting down on smoking and drinking tea and coffee, especially just before bed or when people get up in the night, is another good idea. For a night-time thirst a milky drink is preferable. Trying to relax as much as possible and learning how to cope with troubling thoughts will also help. This is very useful for those times when a person might lie awake with their mind full of distressing thoughts, or if they are kept awake by positive symptoms such as hearing voices.

SEXUAL PROBLEMS

Anyone can suffer sexual problems. However, some of the more common problems for men and women are linked either to specific mental health problems, like anxiety and depression, or can result as an unwanted side effect of psychotropic medication. Neuroleptics can affect virtually all aspects of sexual activity, and it is often these side effects that cause most concern to people who take this medication. The tricyclic antidepressants can cause erectile dysfunction, and new drugs (e.g. Prozac) can cause retarded ejaculation and orgasmic dysfunction. Common sexual problems reported include:

Women

- decreased sexual desire

- impaired sexual arousal

- inability to achieve orgasm.

Men

- decreased sexual desire

- erectile dysfunction

- inability to ejaculate.

When we talk about loss of sexual desire it is important to remember that there is a great amount of normal variation in levels of libido and sexual activity between individuals. We are really concerned with circumstances when a particular person's sexual feelings and behaviour become altered. This need not only involve activity with a partner. Sexual thoughts and fantasies, feelings of attraction to other people and masturbation can be affected.

It is not only medication that can cause difficulties for people's sex lives. The effects of negative symptoms can severely disrupt sexual relationships, or get in the way of establishing these. Depression can also cause people to withdraw, or people can mistakenly feel that they do not deserve affection. People with elevated mood might become involved in unwanted sexual liaisons because of disinhibition. An important component of sexual problems generally can be feelings of anxiety or low self-esteem. The effects of these are often more pronounced in people who have anxiety or depression as features of their illness.

EFFECTS ON RELATIONSHIPS

Relationships can suffer when a person at home has a severe mental health problem. It can be incredibly difficult for families to cope with a person's symptoms and changed behaviours, and the reactions of family members, however well intentioned, can cause added problems for the sufferer. Problems range from the relatively trivial to seemingly unresolvable arguments and conflict. Services can offer help and advice if families are affected in this way. There are also other things that people can do for themselves that may help.

When a person is afflicted by the problems and symptoms of severe mental illness, then it can seem to the people who know them that their whole personality has changed. They may have strange and upsetting symptoms, or they may do things that they never used to. All of this can be very difficult to understand or cope with. Families will usually want to help their relative but may feel unsure or even powerless to know what to do for the best. In these circumstances is is *understandable* if families fall into a pattern of tiredness, irritability and arguments. Another way family members might respond is to become over-protective and attempt to do everything for their relative, in effect taking over responsibility for their life. This might involve self-sacrificing acts like giving up their job, or living very close to somebody, virtually following them around for fear that they may come to harm. These sort of things create stress for everybody and might lead to a person's symptoms or problems getting worse.

It is important to remember that most people do not like tense atmospheres or arguments. If families fall out or argue, or become over-protective, it is because they *care* and are distressed and upset about how things have changed. If the atmosphere at home does become quite emotionally charged, one thing that can happen is that people lose sight of positive things, focusing just on the negative and problematic. This leads to people being hostile and critical to each other, and finding it difficult to solve problems amongst themselves. A way around this is to try and focus on good things that people do or say, and make a point of complimenting them.

The flip side of this is the need to express upsetting or negative feelings. This need does not go away, and it is important not to avoid difficult issues or to try and bottle up feelings. However, if we have to tell somebody that they have upset us or made us feel bad, then we must do this in clear and calm language so that we are not misunderstood. We must also offer people a way of sorting out the issue which has caused us upset. Clearly and calmly letting people know when they have made us feel good or bad can help reduce tensions and stress at home, making it easier to avoid arguments.

Another factor that can cause stress in families is what happens when we ask people to do things. If somebody finds it difficult to get themselves motivated or up and about (types of negative symptoms), it can seem that they are just being lazy or awkward. This leads to people being nagged or pushed into doing things. Of course, it is good to try and keep active but, ideally, a balance needs to be reached where people are encouraged to keep busy not pushed too hard in ways that increase stress. Again, it helps to speak to a person calmly and clearly, saying exactly what it is that we want them to do. It is also useful to explain the positive effects it might have if they do what is asked. For instance, it could make you feel happy or cared for if somebody made you a cup of tea.

An important skill for people to have, especially if they live in difficult circumstances, is to be able to solve problems amongst themselves. An important first step is for everybody to agree what the problem actually is. To achieve this it is crucial that everyone *really* listens to what everyone else has to say. Without this, and some of the other ways of communicating we have looked at, it can be too hard to discuss problems in a group in any meaningful way. However, it is easier to do this if everyone speaks clearly and calmly and listens to others' points of view.

These and other strategies for relieving stress in relationships are the essence of psychosocial approaches and are systematised in **behavioural family therapy**, which we will return to later.

STIGMA

The effects of being exposed to stigma are a sad fact of life for many people with severe mental health problems. However, not everybody has negative views about mental health problems, and people's attitudes generally are improving. When we come across the effects of stigma or people who rely upon it, *they can be challenged and resisted.*

The word 'stigma' describes what happens when people have negative attitudes or beliefs about a certain group of people so that they act towards them in disapproving ways. Some people will think that psychotic problems are strange and frightening and that the people who suffer these problems are very different from themselves. When people do this they are creating an 'identity' for another person, which they assume is accurate, and then apply to all people who they think of as deserving it. The thing about stigma is that the ascribed identity is *always* a 'spoiled' or tainted identity. People who carry stigma are 'marked out' and treated differently from other people.

In this case the 'identity' is applied to all those people 'labelled' as 'mental patients', 'mentally ill' or other even more demeaning labels. These might include 'mad people' or 'nutters' or 'schizos'. Clearly, it is not just individual people who do this. Such inaccurate labels are commonplace in newspapers, on television, in films or most other places you might care to look. The attachment of stigma is a problem of society as a whole.

The important thing to remember about stigma is that the negative ways in which stigmatised people are portrayed in the media, or talked about by other people, are wrong and unfair. It can never be right to talk about a large and diverse group of people as if they are all the same. It is even worse to do this in a way which falsely represents them. When people take up a negative image of mental health this probably says more about them, and their own fears and insecurities, than can be said about the reality of experiencing mental health problems.

Interestingly, many more positive images of people with mental health problems are now being presented by the media. Individuals and pressure groups, such as MIND, can all play their part in offering more accurate information and providing challenges to ignorant people. A good, recent example of how the media can present accurate and generally positive portrayals of schizophrenia has been the depiction of the character 'Joe' and his family in the BBC soap opera *Eastenders*.

Section 2 – Treatment approaches to schizophrenia

Having looked at the characteristics and symptoms of schizophrenia, we now consider treatment approaches. We have already said that the usual treatment for schizophrenia is long-term **medication** (p. 18), which is taken even when symptoms are under control. Other interventions, psychological and social, are also available which address problems such as tolerance to stress, anxiety and depression, as well as other coping difficulties experienced by the patient and family. These involve working with sufferers and other important people, including family, friends and carers, in an attempt to reduce the impact of stress in people's lives.

In this section, physical and psychological treatments are considered in considerable detail in relation to care of schizophrenia. The intention is to develop an appreciation of the value of combining therapeutic approaches to maximise benefit to the patient and family.

NEUROLEPTIC MEDICATION

Within your role you may have direct experience of administering and monitoring medication for patients diagnosed as schizophrenic. This section may be useful in providing more information to help you fulfill this role, or it may serve as a useful revision activity for you if you routinely work with such patients.

The chemical action of neuroleptic medication will be discussed before considering its therapeutic benefits, the adverse effects associated with some drugs used and issues relating to drug therapy, such as patient compliance. You may find it useful when reading this section to have a drug formulary close to hand to look up drugs and terms which are new to you.

Action of neuroleptic drugs

The standard treatment for schiozphrenia is **neuroleptic medication**, a group of compounds originally developed as antihistamines which have been recognised since the early 1950s to have antipsychotic properties (Delay *et al.*, 1952). One of the first drugs of note which was seen to have considerable impact on schizophrenia was chlorpromazine, which you may have heard of or administered at some time.

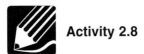 **Activity 2.8**

List other drugs which are classified as neuroleptic. You may be able to do this because of experience of administering them in practice, or you may need to refer to a drug formulary. (Tip: you may need to look under the heading of 'Drugs relating to the central nervous system in general and antipsychotic drugs in particular', Chapter 4 in *British National Formulary*.)

 Feedback to Activity 2.8

In your search you will have found numerous drugs which fall under the heading of neuroleptic or antipsychotic. Common ones used today are:

Drug	Dosage	Administration route
Haloperidol (Serenace)	0.5–2.0 mg bd/tds up to 3.5 mg bd/tds	Oral
Chlorpromazine (Largactil)	10–100 mg tds/qds	Oral

Neuroleptic drugs are active in blocking the uptake of various chemicals, most notably the neurotransmitter **dopamine**, at different receptor sites in the brain. This seems to give credance to a biological explanation for the cause of schizophrenia and psychotic symptoms. These explanations have come to be referred to as the **dopamine hypothesis** (Carlsson and Lindqvuist, 1963). However, with the advent of newer antipsychotic drugs which act at different receptor sites, sometimes involving other neurotransmitters such as **serotonin**, the biochemical explanations for psychosis have had to undergo continual revision.

Evidence from a number of controlled trials indicates that patients taking neuroleptic medication experience less positive symptoms and require fewer hospital admissions because of reduced rates of relapse (Hirsch, 1986) in comparison with those patients not taking any medication. In a recent review of studies concerned with neuroleptic withdrawal, Gilbert *et al.* (1995) found, in a ten-month follow-up period:

- relapse rates of 53% for patients who stopped taking neuroleptic medication

- relapse rates of 16% for those maintained on neuroleptics.

Even though positive and dramatic benefits for the majority of schizophrenic sufferers can be seen, neuroleptic medication is not the answer for everyone; there also exists a group of sufferers – up to 40% – who continue to experience some degree of psychotic problems, often referred to as **residual symptoms**, even when taking prescribed medication. This group who remain symptomatic can be described as **treatment resistant** or **therapy refractory**. However, there is a growing body of evidence that the newer, **atypical** neuroleptics are effective in these circumstances (Lindstrom and Wieselgren, 1996). The therapeutic blockade of brain chemistry can also have unwanted neurological and physical **side effects** resulting in varying degrees of distress, commonly leading to an unwillingness to continue taking the medication.

Neuroleptics are seen to be most effective against relapse in instances where individuals may be viewed as being particularly vulnerable to such stress and are exposed to various psychosocial stressors. Medication is not perhaps indicated for those who do not face a stressful environment or are not having to cope with stressful life events. This case has been most strongly made by Johnstone (1993) in observing the relatively constant and low relapse rates in low **expressed emotion** households, whether a person is taking neuroleptic medication or not. (We shall consider the nature of expressed emotion and its relevance to schizophrenia later in the book.) However, this view is challenged by the overwhelming majority of interested commentators, who recommend various prescribing strategies aimed at maximising therapeutic benefit whilst encouraging patient compliance in taking the prescribed medication. This usually involves balancing psychotic symptoms and levels of social functioning against the potential impact of side effects, at the lowest manageable dose. Kane and Marder (1993) found that relatively low doses of neuroleptics are as clinically effective as higher doses, but induce less side effects and reduce adverse impact upon social functioning. A recent meta-analysis of randomised controlled trials supports such a minimum therapeutic dose approach. It found that above a certain dose (equivalent to 375 mg chlorpromazine) there was no reported incremental improvement in symptom alleviation (Bollini *et al.*, 1994).

It is important for us to realise that neuroleptics do not provide a cure for schizophrenia, and the responses of individuals to specific neuroleptic drugs or differing dosages of the same drug are variable and therefore may be difficult to predict. A further complicating factor is the considerable variation of blood plasma uptake of neuroleptics across individuals (Silverstone and Turner, 1991). As you may already know through experience, individual responsiveness to drugs may also be influenced by such factors as age, body weight, physical constitution and diet – including alcohol, caffeine and nicotine consumption (Hubbard *et al.*, 1993). It has also been demonstrated that people who do not respond to a particular neuroleptic never will, and the prescription ought to be changed (Brown and Herz, 1989). In practice, neuroleptic prescribing ought to proceed in a stepwise fashion, with differing compounds being tried out in turn for efficacy. For patients and their families this can seem at best somewhat 'hit and miss', or at worst totally arbitrary.

Side effects associated with neuroleptics

We have already said that therapeutic responses to neuroleptics are variable and difficult to predict. Similarly, the presence of side effects, which are usually related to dosage, is also variable and idiosyncratic. The different forms of receptor blockade provided by the different sub-types of neuroleptics cause particular groupings of side effects; however, all neuroleptics can produce a well-defined range of side effects to one extent or another.

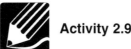 **Activity 2.9**

Think about patients within your caseload. Make a list of those side effects which are commonly presented in individuals taking neuroleptic drugs. Alternatively, read about such effects in your formulary and list the most common ones. Consider patients' thoughts and feelings in response to experiencing such side effects.

Feedback to Activity 2.9

As you will have realised, there is quite a range of side effects which commonly occur. Specific neuroleptic side effects include:

- **sedation**: all neuroleptics result in some degree of sedation, particularly at high doses.

- **extrapyramidal symptoms**: these are neurological effects which impact upon voluntary muscle movement, posture and coordination. There are four main types of extrapyramidal effect:

  1 **parkinsonian symptoms** – drug-induced effects which are indistinguishable from the symptoms of Parkinson's disease, e.g. problems with gait, expressionless facial appearance, tremor, rigidity, slowness of movement, difficulty swallowing. These effects are reversible with anticholinergic medication, e.g. procyclidine.

  2 **dystonia** – muscle spasms, usually of the face and neck, which can result in people's bodies contorting into unnatural postures. This can happen to the muscles which control the eyes, causing a fixed upward stare referred to as **oculogyric crisis**. These side effects are more common in younger people and can be very distressing, though they are rapidly resolved with intramuscular or intravenous injection of an anticholinergic.

  3 **akathisia** – an inner feeling of restlessness, sometimes accompanied by restless movements such as pacing, rocking or an inability to sit down in one place. Because these effects can be misinterpreted as an exacerbation of psychotic symptoms, they can be exacerbated by inappropriate increases in prescribed medication.

  4 **tardive dyskinesia** – involuntary, repetitive movements of the tongue and mouth. These usually develop in older people, being more common in women, and can be irreversible. There is no known remedy and the problem can be worsened by withdrawing neuroleptic treatment.

- **anticholinergic effects**:

  - dry mouth

  - nausea or vomitting

  - constipation

  - blurred vision

  - urinary retention or difficulties with micturition.

- **cardiovascular effects**:

  - most commonly, dizziness or fainting when arising from a chair, getting out of bed or leaving a hot bath, resulting from **postural hypotension**

  - the risk of cardiac arryhthmia can be 10 times greater than that for the general population.

- **weight gain**: a common effect, but usually mild increases in weight. However, some patients can gain as much as two or three stones. Such a scenario can be exacerbated by inactivity, itself a not uncommon feature of such people's lives.

- **skin sensitivity reactions**:
  - rashes – itchy or dry skin. These can also affect practitioners who come into contact with liquid neuroleptic preparations
  - photosensitivity – particularly associated with chlorpromazine, so greatly increased susceptibility to sunburn.

- **sexual side effects**:
  - reduced libido
  - orgasmic dysfunction
  - erectile dysfunction, including priapism
  - ejaculatory dysfunction
  - amenorrhoea
  - gynaecomastia and galactorrhoea, occurring in both women and men.

- **agranulocytosis**: potentially fatal blood disorder (30% mortality rate) which occurs very rarely as a consequence of most neuroleptic medication. However, the incidence is relatively higher (between 1–2 in every 100) for those prescribed **clozapine**, and for this reason use of this drug is always accompanied by rigorous blood testing.

- **jaundice**: can occur as an allergic reaction in the first few weeks of commencing treatment with **phenothiazine** neuroleptics, e.g. chlorpromazine. Requires discontinuation of the particular neuroleptic.

- **neuroleptic malignant syndrome**: a serious, life-threatening complication of neuroleptic therapy in between 0.5 and 1% of clients. It is more usually associated with high-potency neuroleptics, and the mortality rate is 20%. The characteristic symptoms of muscular rigidity, pyrexia, fluctuating consciousness, rapid pulse and sweating can be mistaken for signs of infection, leading to ineffective treatment. Once diagnosed, discontinuation of neuroleptic treatment and transfer to an intensive care unit is recommended. Because the condition can persist for some time after stopping the drug, this is complicated if a **depot** preparation has been used.

 You may wish to explore further the side effects relating to neuroleptics. A useful source of information is Bazire's pocket guide *GP Psychotropic Handbook*, which is published annually (Bazire, 1998). Within your practice you can assess the frequency and severity of particular side effects for individuals by using the self-report Liverpool University Side Effects Rating Scale (LUNSERS) (Day *et al.*, 1995).

Adherence to prescribed medication

There are a number of factors that can adversely influence the extent to which people comply with programmes of neuroleptic medication. In your response to the last activity you may have identified that some patients find

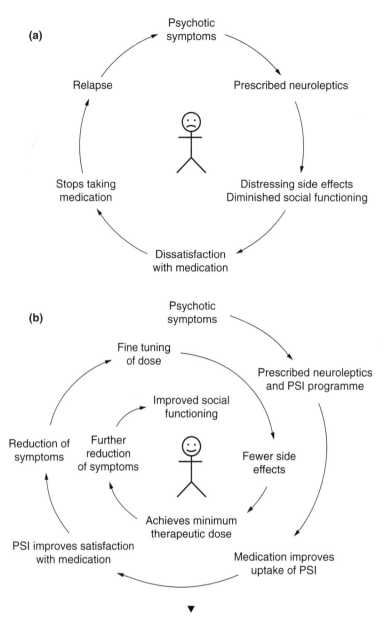

**Figure 2.2 Improving adherence to prescribed medication:
(a) Vicious circle; (b) Virtuous circle.**

the side effects to be inconvenient or uncomfortable. **The most obvious
reason for refusing to take medication is a reaction to the distress
caused by side effects**. To some extent this situation can be improved
by informing people of the possibility of side effects before taking the
medication. Negative experiences of unscientific prescribing practices, such
as multiple prescribing or too high dosages, can also have a detrimental
impact upon compliance. Confusion, disorientation or suspicion, particularly
when people are relatively unwell, can all contribute to failures to take
medication as directed. Figure 2.2a illustrates the vicious circle which
results when an individual stops taking medication. Relapse, readmission
and prolonged distress can often result due to lack of informed compliance
to the medication programme prescribed. Figure 2.2b illustrates how an
educational element – to give information about benefits and side effects of

medication – breaks the vicious circle and involves the patient in a virtuous circle where symptoms are managed, and where relapse and distress is minimised.

It is for these reasons that neuroleptics are often prescribed in an injectable, slow-release form, called depot medication, which ensures a consistent dose over a set time. Another advantage is that the administration of depot medication is a convenient means for patients to keep some contact with services, which prevents isolation and helps early detection of relapse. Conversely, depot medication has been criticised because of the implied lack of trust in clients, the denial of individual responsibility and overtones of social control.

The optimum therapeutic alliance is achieved when well-targeted medication enables the patient to be amenable to other interventions such as PSI. This amenability takes the form of improved motivation and more rational thinking, which enables uptake of psychosocial therapies. This, in turn, helps to improve adherence to prescribed medication, allowing for collaborative fine-tuning of dosage towards minimum therapeutic levels, thus minimising side effects, in a '**virtuous circle**' of patient improvement.

Therapeutic optimism

Given the promising results of research into PSI and the developments in new atypical neuroleptics, there are grounds for contemplating a brighter future in the treatment of schizophrenia. Though it must be acknowledged that medication does not cure schizophrenia, most of the recent research into treatment suggests grounds for optimism in relation to better outcomes. Well-targeted combinations of neuroleptic treatment and PSI would seem to be the most beneficial approach, especially in the early stages of the disorder (Lindstrom and Wieselgren, 1996).

THE PSYCHOLOGICAL MANAGEMENT OF SYMPTOMS

There is a growing body of work which evaluates the effectiveness of a range of psychological interventions for the management of symptoms in schizophrenic individuals. These interventions are important because of the fact that many people, even those who are relatively well on medication, still experience residual symptoms. Psychological approaches may become the primary intervention for those people who cannot or will not take medication, usually because of excessive or distressing side effects. Most of the techniques found to be useful are **behavioural** or, more latterly, **cognitive-behavioural** approaches. Some aim to build upon the fact that people who experience psychotic problems will invariably have tested out their own self-help management techniques, leading to the therapy tactic of **coping strategy enhancement**.

The research studies

Various research studies have attempted to evaluate these psychological interventions for psychosis in clinical practice. Until recently most of these studies were small-scale or even single case study designs, but more recently they have been subject to more rigorous scrutiny in a number of controlled trials, with others underway. Most of the research has focused specifically on positive symptoms, notably delusions and auditory hallucinations. Some have attempted to demonstrate an impact on the negative symptoms of schizophrenia, particularly attention, memory and the problem-solving abilities of patients. The development and furtherance of this significant body of research and implementation in clinical practice ought to realise important benefits in the community management of schizophrenia.

 Several comprehensive reviews of the literature in this area of clinical research are in print (Slade, 1990; Birchwood and Shepherd, 1992; Tarrier, 1992; Bentall *et al.*, 1994), providing an overview of the different methods of psychological intervention which have been undertaken. An important text is *Cognitive-Behavioural Interventions with Psychotic Disorders* (Haddock and Slade, 1996) which features a number of key practitioners and researchers who discuss their work in the context of case examples, and argue for the integration of these methods into clinical practice to support other psychosocial approaches.

A wide range of particular interventions, geared towards the improvement of specific symptoms, have been described. Given the complexity and diversity of symptoms and problems both between and within individuals, it is not surprising that the research tends to demonstrate that *some* of these interventions seem to work for *some* people. That is, these psychological techniques must not be seen as some sort of panacea, and different approaches might need to be tried with individuals until a successful method is hit upon. However, the burgeoning research into this field of clinical practice would suggest optimism for the development of both effective therapies and more sophisticated understandings of relevant psychological processes associated with psychotic symptoms. In the long run this may lead to much improved targeting of psychological interventions.

It is not possible to recount all of the relevant research in detail, but those psychological methods which have been found to be useful for specific symptom groups are now listed and discussed briefly.

Positive symptoms

Hallucinations

- **operant procedures** – rewarding changes in behaviour which reduce hallucinations (Nydegger, 1972)

- **systematic desensitisation** – assessing those stressors which contribute to or make hallucinations worse, then reducing them (Slade, 1972)

- **thought stopping** – actively stopping hallucinations by telling them to stop or mentally switching them off (Johnson *et al.*, 1983)

- **distraction** – using the radio or a Walkman to distract the person's thoughts away from their hallucinations. Similarly, a person might attempt to distract themselves from voices by reading, doing mental arithmetic or playing mental games (Margo *et al.*, 1981; James, 1983; Nelson *et al.*, 1991; Gallagher *et al.*, 1994)

- **self-monitoring** – a therapy in itself, by helping the person to recognise when and how often they experience hallucinations. May involve keeping a diary (Reybee and Kinch, 1973, unpublished, cited in Slade, 1990)

- **ear plugs** – using ear plugs in left or right ear to reduce auditory hallucinations (James, 1983)

- **first person singular therapy** – teaching people to reject the view that they have no control at all over their hallucinations (Greene, 1978)

- **focusing and reattribution approach** – teaching people to focus attention on the various features of their hallucinations, like loudness or frequency, especially the meanings these symptoms hold in people's lives; modifying beliefs, for instance about where the voices come from (Haddock and Slade, 1996)

Slade and Bentall (1988) suggest that much that has been found of use in psychologically treating hallucinations can be incorporated into one of three categories:

1 those that emphasise distraction

2 those that encourage patients to focus on their voices

3 those that involve anxiety reduction.

Distraction techniques generally aim to encourage patients to divert their attention away from their hallucinations. This can involve passive distraction (such as using a radio or Walkman), active internal distraction (such as reading or mental arithmetic) or active external distraction (such as reading aloud, humming or whistling). Some of these distraction methods are thought to work because of a view which sees auditory hallucinations as a misattribution of internal events to the external world. In essence, hallucinatory voices are thought to be misperceived internal voices, like those ways of talking to ourselves that everybody has. There is some evidence for this hypothesis in the phenomenon of **sub-vocal speech**. It has been observed that when anybody thinks to themselves there is activity in the region of the vocal chords. This sub-vocal activity is replicated in voice-hearing subjects. Distraction therapies such as reading out loud can be seen as an attempt to use the vocal chords in another way; for this reason these distraction approaches are also referred to as **counterstimulation**.

Misattributing an internally generated voice as an external voice suggests the possibility of working with people to **reattribute** the perceived source of their voices, or other beliefs they have acquired them about. This has usually been accomplished within a form of therapy which involves **focusing** as a first step. Focusing aims to help the person examine closely the content of their hallucinations, their subjective meaning and the person's beliefs and assumptions about their experiences. These beliefs are then modified to reduce the distress and, hopefully, frequency of voices. People are taught how to pay attention to the content of what their voices say and focus upon the characteristics of the voice, for instance the volume, pitch and tone, or whether it is of a recognised person. By exploring the relationship between the voice and what is said, and the voice hearer and their life, it is possible to attempt some changes.

Anxiety reduction utilises the patient's environment and their responses to that environment as areas to modify, thereby reducing their hallucinations.

As can be seen, there are a number of ways of helping people who are distressed or have their lives disrupted by hearing voices. Many people may have learnt to use some of these by their own experimentation with self-coping strategies, which may be more or less helpful. Hence the use of earplugs or Walkmans is quite common, without people having had to attend structured therapy sessions. Other people have found that they can cope better either by ignoring their voices, concentrating on listening to them, telling the voices to go away or reaching 'an agreement' with the voices that they will only be listened to at a certain time of the day. Relaxation exercises help some people, whilst others rely on changes to their diet. All of these approaches, and there are many more, have been found to help *some* people to a greater or lesser degree, but may not work for others.

Many of these themes have been taken up by the group 'Hearing Voices', an international self-help network. The **Hearing Voices Network** has local branches, distributes a newsletter and other literature, and holds conferences. The main thrust of the group is to accept voices as real and meaningful, promoting the use of *effective* therapies *only* when the voices cause distress. These issues and themes are discussed at length in the excellent text from the co-founders of the Hearing Voices movement, Marius Romme and Sandra Escher, *Accepting Voices* (1993).

Delusions

- **operant procedures** – rewarding non-delusional speech so people talk about their delusions less (Liberman *et al.*, 1973)

- **belief modification** – challenging the evidence for certain beliefs rather than directly challenging the belief itself (Watts *et al.*, 1973; Chadwick and Lowe, 1990)

- **reality testing** – setting up small practical 'experiments' wherein the outcome serves to challenge the basis for delusional beliefs (Chadwick and Lowe, 1990)

Behavioural or operant approaches can help people to limit the extent to which they talk to other people about their delusions. This can help if the beliefs are likely to seem strange to other people, avoiding adverse reactions or embarrassment.

Belief modification is interesting because the approach relies on a **cognitive model** of *all beliefs*, thus demonstrating how *everybody* acts upon information from their environment in ways which are influenced by what they believe, regardless of the actual content of specific beliefs (see Bentall, 1996, p. 12). It would be much too time-consuming for people to

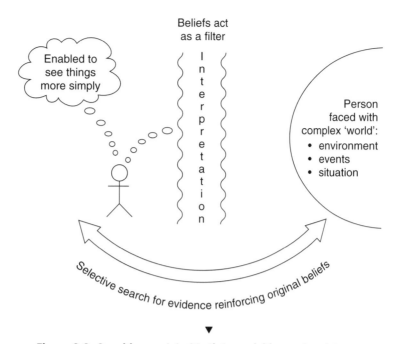

Figure 2.3 Cognitive model of belief acquisition and maintenance.

stop and ask questions of all the day-to-day events and circumstances with which they may be faced before they make decisions about how to act. Indeed, we are usually quite unaware that any decision-making process has gone on at all for most everyday occurrences that we come across. But, if we think about it, even seemingly trivial events or interactions can be quite complex in reality. One of the psychological techniques that people have developed to help them negotiate life in a complicated world is to use their beliefs and attitudes to help them quickly make inferences or assumptions about the situations they find themselves in. In this sense, our beliefs act as a *filter* on the world, allowing us to *interpret* what is going on – in essence, simplifying matters. This process is complicated by another psychological knack that we have of searching our environment for new information, often doing this *selectively* in a way which *provides evidence supportive of the original belief*. This model is represented diagramatically in Figure 2.3.

Essentially, we look for evidence which confirms what we believe and tend to ignore evidence which does not support this view. You only need to think of the damaging effects of stereotypes about minorities to see this in action. In these instances assumptions are made about large, heterogenous groups of people such that they become homogenised in narrow and unwholesome ways. A less extreme example is the Everton supporter who can see no wrong in his team! Of course, all our beliefs and attitudes work this way, without us giving them too much thought, and usually this helps us to manage our lives quite well. This process has probably developed because of the evolutionary value in being able to make snap decisions around personal safety. Think about the cave dweller faced with a sabre-toothed tiger. In this scenario you do not want to interrogate the situation before making a decision what to do. You would assume danger, and leave quickly!

When a person holds a delusional belief this will also operate as a filter on the world, perhaps causing problems. A person who is paranoid will interpret events in ways that support a belief that people are out to do them harm. You may have seen the episode of *Eastenders* where *Joe*, the schizophrenic character, sees some workers digging up the road and interprets this as an attempt to tunnel into his flat. Hence confirming his belief that people were 'out to get' him and his dad. Interestingly, in the same episode, Joe's dad, *David Wicks*, is accused of trying to kidnap the child of *Ian Beale*, a character who has already had two of his children taken away by their mother with the assistance of *David*, who had been having an affair with her. In reality, *David* had merely found the child who had wandered away from her dad in a crowded marketplace. However, because *Ian* had suspicions about *David*, and was fearful he would lose his other child, when he saw her with *David* he interpreted this as an abduction in process, rather than an attempt to return the child. The ensuing altercation was further proof for *Joe* that people were set against him and his father. Such is the stuff of soap opera scripts, but a nonetheless useful illustration of cognitive processes in action.

Some of the most effective therapies for delusions attempt to work around the sort of mental processes described above. A cognitive-behavioural strategy tries to help a person to challenge the 'evidence' they have for their belief. It is not thought to be helpful to directly or forcibly challenge the core belief itself. However, by providing alternative and plausible explanations for the reasons people offer in support of their belief, then, in time, the extent to which people firmly believe the delusion can begin to be shaken. Such approaches are best undertaken systematically by trained therapists, but friends and family can try to understand delusions in this way so that they can learn to say helpful things in conversation.

Chadwick and Lowe (1990) describe how they modified the delusions of some clients using structured verbal challenge and reality testing of their beliefs. Prior to any intervention they comprehensively assessed the person's conviction and preoccupation with their belief. They then assessed the evidence which had helped the person establish their belief and asked them to rank the evidence in order of importance. This baseline assessment preceeded a structured, verbal challenge of each piece of evidence supporting the delusion, commencing with the least important. Throughout, the interviewer took a non-confrontational stance, merely putting forward alternative interpretations to events. Following this verbal challenge, some subjects were then asked to test out their belief in reality, with the therapist, to prove or disprove their belief. Results showed a marked decrease in conviction and preoccupation with delusions in five out of the six subjects.

Coping strategy enhancement

Systematic and flexible packages of enhancing coping strategies have been developed to assist people to manage the distress of both hallucinations and delusions. In the UK this work has been largely associated with Nick Tarrier and colleagues (see Tarrier, 1992; Tarrier *et al.*, 1990). The **coping strategy enhancement** approach works at building individualised training programmes in appropriate behavioural and cognitive methods of coping, which aim to supplement and advance the sort of self-help coping strategies which individuals have developed for themselves as a means of reducing their own symptoms or the associated distress.

This approach has been evaluated in comparison to structured **problem solving** using controlled study:

- One group involved the enhancement of coping strategies by assessing the subjects' own strategies, practising them within sessions and then applying that strategy in a structured, consistent way. Other strategies were then selected for other symptoms and applied systematically.

- The second group involved learning problem-solving strategies and applying this method to real-life situations.

Results demonstrated that patients in both groups showed significant improvements in symptom-related assessments. Further, that patients in the coping strategy enhancement group improved more than patients in the problem-solving group. However, there was little improvement in social functioning or negative symptoms.

Thought disorder

Thought linkage and clarification – attempts to make sense of illogical and incoherent speech (Kingdon and Turkington, 1991).

It is possible to get help for thought disorder, or, importantly, for other people to help. Most of the innovative work being initiated in this respect is based upon the work of David Kingdon and Douglas Turkington (for a brief exposition of their approach see their 1995 book *Cognitive-behavior Therapy of Schizophrenia*, pp. 146–8). Such approaches demand a lot of time and patience. It is particularly important to listen to what people say, however difficult it is to make sense of. However disordered a person's speech might be, it is usually possible to pick out something from the jumble. Therapists who have studied these problems suggest that it is best to look for themes which seem to run through the conversation, and to begin to talk about these. Eventually, after a lot of perseverance on both sides, some meanings might become clearer.

An important first step might be for a person to try and slow down their speech, or for other people to help them to do this. A skilled therapist tries to move towards hitting upon bits of the conversation or single words upon which they can agree the meaning. They might suggest other words to use for the same meaning, to make the speech easier to understand for other people. The therapist works in stages of listening, stopping, rephrasing, checking accuracy of meaning, discussion, agreement, restarting and continued listening, until the whole speech becomes gradually more coherent. Family and friends can help with this process, particularly if there are differences in the use of language between the therapist and the person with speech problems. For instance the person might have a strong regional accent or English might be a second language. It is always the case that friends and family will know a person's normal speech better. Other strategies might be used to improve attention and concentration skills.

Negative symptoms

- **token economy** – gaining positive rewards for certain behaviours (Ayllon and Azrin, 1968)

- **social skills training** – the improvement of carefully assessed functional deficits (Hogarty *et al.*, 1986)

- **problem solving** – training given in the planning and implementation of problem-solving skills (Hansen *et al.*, 1985)

- **cognitive rehabilitation** – (Goldberg and Triano-Antidormi, 1992)

Reports of improvements in negative symptoms using psychological interventions are relatively thin on the ground. Programmes such as **token economy** and **social skills training** tend to encompass a series of interventions or a rehabilitation package which aims to affect lifestyles rather than specific symptoms. One such package which appears to be demonstrating benefits is that described by Goldberg and Triano-Antidormi (1992). This programme attempts to address social functioning deficits which result from problems with the client's memory, attention and problem solving. Interventions consist of three main approaches which they term **cognitive rehabilitation**:

1 **adjustment to loss** – this involves changing the person's environment to compensate for any cognitive deficits. An example would be limiting vocational placements or therapy to short periods with long breaks so as to aid attention difficulties.

2 **strategy building** – this involves the use of coping devices which will help the patient live as independently as possible. An example of this might be the use of a daily planner to aid in structuring the day, or the use of memos or cards to aid in planning behaviour.

3 **cognitive retraining** – this is the training or recovering of impaired cognitive skills through practice. A particular training package is the Attention Process Training (APT) pack, developed by Sohlberg and Mateer (1989). This uses audio and visual exercises which aim to practise and develop attentional skills and memory.

Goldberg and Triano-Antidormi (1992) in summary state that although the research programme is in its infancy, promising results have already been achieved in improving attention in clients with schizophrenia.

Application of psychological and cognitive interventions to practice

Perhaps the most attractive element of these psychological interventions must be in their empowering and enabling nature. They are not treatments imposed on patients with or without their consent – they are client-focused, collaborative ventures which aim to acknowledge and build upon the coping strategies already available to the person. The basis for all of this work is in developing more control by the patient over their experiences. It is more about identifying real strategies for coping rather than merely applying more physical treatments which research has shown are not fully effective against persistent symptoms (Kingdon *et al.*, 1994). Importantly, there is an underlying philosophy of **normalising** unusual experiences and paying attention to psychotic symptoms in terms of their **meaningfulness** to people and the **roles** they assume within their lives. In many respects this advance in therapy is a massive contradiction to what had previously been taught to novice practitioners. The edict not to talk or listen to people's 'crazy' beliefs or accounts of their strange experiences, for fear of 'collusion' or making these problems worse, has been replaced by a new openness and reflexivity where talking about and engaging with psychotic experiences *is the therapy*. Of course, schizophrenia sufferers have probably always known this, and individuals will remember the people who attempt to listen to them in times of illness and distress.

It is clear that recent research into the application of psychological interventions in the management of schizophrenia has demonstrated many benefits. Studies have shown that clients can be enabled to gain more control over their symptoms, improve their social functioning, reduce distress and raise attention and problem-solving ability. Moreover, the research challenges conventional beliefs about delusions and hallucinations. They demonstrate that they are amenable to reasoning approaches, provided they are challenged in a non-confrontational and collaborative way (Kingdon *et al.*, 1994).

A healthy criticism of these approaches and further research is needed if we are to be able to identify which are the most applicable to which symptoms and how benefits can be generalised into social functioning. Enough evidence has been collated, however, to give credence to the approaches being applied in clinical practice by appropriately knowledgeable and skilled practitioners.

Section 3 – Prevention of relapse

Up to now we have considered active treatment approaches for the individual with schizophrenia. It is important to ensure that, once restored to optimum levels of functioning, the patient is assisted, as far as the course of his condition will allow, to maintain that 'healthy state'. To do so requires some careful monitoring and therapeutic inputs to prevent relapse, or to detect early relapse and to prevent serious breakdown. In this section we will consider early warning signs and discuss the role of the mental health services.

In schizophrenia, people may have a pattern of illness which involves repeated episodes. The person might be completely well, or have few symptoms in between episodes, but from time to time becomes unwell. The periods of acute illness are referred to as relapses. Relapses themselves are distressing for both the schizophrenia sufferer and their family. It is also thought that the frequency with which a person relapses might have an overall negative effect upon a person's long-term mental health. It may be the case that even though people can make a recovery between relapses, there is a cumulative trend towards deterioration such that people do not quite recover to their pre-relapse state of functioning each time. For these reasons it is important to try and avoid relapses.

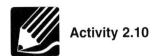 **Activity 2.10**

What interventions could help prevent relapse? List helpful behaviours that the patient could adopt to maintain health.

 Feedback to Activity 2.10

A variety of behaviours may minimise relapse. Some general ways to try and avoid relapse include:

- long-term use of medication

- learning to manage and cope with stress

- working together with family and friends on ways of communicating needs and feelings, and how problems are solved at home

- looking after physical health

- keeping in touch with healthcare staff

- keeping active socially or at work, but balancing this against pressure and stress.

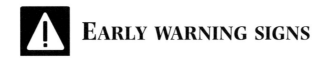 # EARLY WARNING SIGNS

An important way of helping to avoid relapse is for the person themselves, their family or professional carers to look out for '**early warning signs**' that a relapse might be about to happen. These early warning signs might be less severe versions of the full-blown symptoms a person has when they are ill, or they might be more vague sensations, thoughts or feelings. The important thing is that they are *typically* what a person experiences just before a relapse, and can be recognised as such. Family, friends and care staff can help to identify early warning signs and work out an action plan to use in the event of these occurring. These early warning signs are also called '**prodromes**' or '**prodromal signs**'. A specific individual's set of warning signs is known as their '**prodromal signature**'. Much of the UK research into monitoring early warning signs has been carried out by Birchwood and colleagues, who provide a staged approach to relapse intervention in *Innovations in the Psychological Management of Schizophrenia* (1992).

Not every person will have, or be able to recognise easily, a clear set of early warning signs. For those that do it is important to remember that they will be very individual, probably unique to them. Having said this, there may be various common features amongst different people's prodromes.

 Activity 2.11

Think about one of your patients who is diagnosed as schizophrenic but who is fairly stable in health terms. Now make a list of possible changes in behaviour which may lead you to be concerned that he/she is beginning to deteriorate from a well state.

Your list should be specific to one particular patient. As stated previously, presenting problems and symptoms may vary from one individual to the next. However, common prodromal signs might include:

- spending more time alone in bedroom

- becoming more irritable, perhaps with specific people

- a particular idea keeps entering a person's thoughts

- fear of going mad

- poor appetite

- low mood

- sleep problems

- certain objects or people seem to assume a special significance or meaning

- thoughts racing

- laughing out loud for no apparent reason.

Birchwood *et al.* (1992) suggest that many of these early warning signs and associated psychological responses by the patient are attempts to find meaning or control over disordered experiences. It is exactly this meaning and control which psychological interventions attempt to provide, hence their relevance and importance. It is clear that people use psychological strategies themselves to cope with symptoms, particularly prior to relapse.

EARLY INTERVENTIONS

It may be useful to identify an individual's warning signs when they are well, so that if any of these signs occur something can be done to try to prevent a full relapse from happening. Early interventions might include:

- adjusting medication

- crisis counselling

- support with stress management and relaxation

- involvement of family and friends

- identifying specific stressors and working on how to cope

- avoiding whatever is causing too much stress at this time

- enhancement of general coping strategies.

Once the early warning signs have been identified, these can be written down and kept handy, but safe. Better still they ought to be discussed and generated in conjunction with the care team and recorded in case notes. This is the sort of information which a person could carry around as part of a crisis card.

Crisis cards

A crisis card is useful for carrying information which might be helpful if, for instance, a person needs to be admitted to hospital, or gets into some sort of trouble. It should include details of identification and what sort of problems have occasioned treatment in the past. The information carried can help schizophrenia sufferers to remind themselves of things, particularly when they might be becoming unwell and are not thinking too clearly. It is also useful for close friends and family, so that they are best informed how to help. For example, early warning signs are recorded in detail, together with which treatments or interventions work best to avoid relapse. If a person is relapsing, the card carries information which tells professional care staff, particularly in a hospital or accident and emergency department where they are not known, how best to help. For instance, the card might record the sort of medication and dose which has been found to be of most therapeutic benefit, whilst noting those which have not helped and are not worth repeating. It should be the person's own decision to carry such a card, only doing so if they think it is a good idea.

 Activity 2.12

Reflect upon what you have read about techniques for reducing or helping with psychotic symptoms. In what ways might your practice incorporate some of these strategies?

Interventions which you thought useful might include:

- **raising insight through education and discussion** – this may involve group or individual discussions involving patients and their families, or with colleagues

- **encouraging patients to self-monitor their symptoms** – strategies to enable patients to monitor accurately their psychotic experiences

- **helping patients and their families to be aware of and monitor prodromal signs** – this identification of 'early warning signs' can enable people to take action before a relapse develops

- **systematically evaluating the patients' own coping mechanisms** – all patients are already coping to some extent with their symptoms, and some are coping very well indeed. By assessing what works for patients and applying those techniques systematically, patients can cope with many distressing symptoms

- **the use of stress management strategies** – by enabling patients to recognise what makes them stressed, and reducing the effects of stress, symptoms can be reduced

- **the involvement of families and friends in effective problem solving** – the ability to solve problems and hence reduce a build-up of stress is important. Training in problem-solving skills enables this

- **provision of or referral for cognitive-behavioural therapy which focuses upon positive symptoms** – specific strategies have been shown to be effective with many symptoms of schizophrenia.

Section 4 – Case management

Whatever the treatment approaches used, the context of care needs to be considered. Over the past ten years the rehabilitation of those with serious mental health needs has been reinforced by a move towards more community care. Many large psychiatric institutions have been and continue to be closed down, with their patients moving into community-based programmes (Moxley, 1989). This large-scale move into the community has created major service delivery problems, particularly with the move to have a primary care-focused National Health Service. Within the community there are now large numbers of clients with multiple mental health needs requiring services which are geographically dispersed, decentralised and fragmented. The monitoring of costs and service duplication has become difficult, if not impossible, which has fueled criticism and led Anthony *et al.* (1983) to comment 'the nightmare of institutionalism has now been replaced by the horrors of deinstitutionalism'.

Case management and the care programme approaches have therefore developed as service system responses to enable the coordination of care (Huxley, 1993). More cynically, case management has become an administrative tool for cost management (Walker, 1982), with case managers establishing eligibility for services rather than assessing needs and strengths (Onyett and Cambridge, 1992). How are services to manage this burden of care and on what principles and methods are they to be organised?

In the United States, where case management has a much longer history, several models of good practice have developed. One model with a long history of use in the US is the psychiatric rehabilitation model. This is designed to develop the client's skills and strengths, whilst at the same time increasing the environmental supports to enable the client to function within the community (Anthony, 1993). Another model, developed in Hamilton, Ontario, focuses on the long-term effects of clients with schizophrenia. This initiative resulted from high admission rates to the behavioural unit and added resources into their community services. The result was a programme which emphasised the complex needs of schizophrenia sufferers and their **assessment**, the need for **continuity of care** across discipline boundaries, **comprehensiveness** of the services available and **coordination**.

Huxley (1993) also defines the core tasks of any model as being assessment of needs and strengths, individual service planning that has clearly defined outcomes, implementation, monitoring and reviewing. Onyett and Cambridge (1992) go further in their review of models of case management and attempt to define which aspects of the various models appear to be most effective. They summarise their ideal model as having a team deliver case management; with peer-reviewed specialist direct input by autonomous practitioners; with micro budgets for buying in direct care for clients, following comprehensive, multidisciplinary assessment by Case Managers who are separate from provision. They also emphasise user-centred services, enabling clients to plan their own programmes.

Definitions of case management (and the case manager role) are clearly numerous, as are the models that describe its implementation. Weil and Karls (1985) insist that services are provided in 'a supportive, effective, efficient and cost-effective manner', while Rothman (1991) expands on these principles, adding its core functions of 'assessment, care planning, direct and indirect intervention, monitoring, review and evaluation'. It is these core functions that appear to be necessary in planning and delivering care to the severely mentally ill.

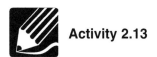 **Activity 2.13**

You have been designated as a case manager for a patient. What would you identify as the responsibilities of that role? You may wish to discuss this with colleagues or actual patients in order to help build up a role description.

Feedback to Activity 2.13

In most models the **case manager role** is crucial in the effective delivery of services. Huxley (1993) identifies several key elements of this important role. The nature of the role of the case manager is one of **brokerage**, where you, as the case manager, would work on behalf of your clients to improve the services available. There may be little, if any, direct input to the client but rather more emphasis being placed on the coordination of others to meet need. Improvement of services and coordination could involve:

- **assessment** of individual needs

- **monitoring** of service delivery and impact of care

- **advocacy** on behalf of patients and family

- **assertive outreach** – the identification of clients by some case managers. The seriously mentally ill may not always be in a position to refer themselves to the services available, so the role of the case manager becomes more intensive, direct and rapid

- the **linkage** role of the case manager in which the manager allocates resources based on the assessments made by other professionals. To enable resource allocation the case manager needs some degree of **budgetary control** in order to match need to services available (Onyett and Cambridge, 1992).

These identified factors inherent in the case manager role need to remain flexible and tailored to individual demands (Weil and Karls, 1985).

Section 5 – The impact of stress in relation to schizophrenia

STRESS IN FAMILY ENVIRONMENTS

In this section we consider the nature and impact of stress within family environments in relation to the individual with schizophrenia. Considering the research will help you to gain an understanding of the rationale for using PSI. Several controlled studies are briefly reviewed, as are a number of other clinical studies, which have implemented and evaluated a variety of programmes. The research projects have generated a great deal of interest as they demonstrate many tangible benefits of PSI in the management of schizophrenia, and may yet provide further methods to improve the lives of carers and sufferers.

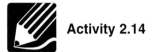 **Activity 2.14**

Before considering the nature of stress which may arise within a family of an individual suffering from schizophrenia, it may be useful first to put yourself in their shoes. Consider the following scenario.

Robert is your close relative living within your household. He is about to be discharged from hospital after being an in-patient for six months. He has been diagnosed as suffering from schizophrenia and has shown a range of distressing symptoms, including hallucinations and delusions (you may wish to refer back to Section 1 of this chapter to remind yourself what these symptoms are). Compulsory admission into hospital was necessary and events leading up to admission were very difficult for you and your family.

- What may your reaction be to him now?

- What practical difficulties could you anticipate after he returns home?

- What have you told or will you tell your friends and neighbours about Robert?

- What help should Robert expect of you?

- What signs would you look for to suggest that Robert is becoming unwell again, and how may you monitor his behaviour?

Feedback to Activity 2.14

You may have direct experience of caring for a schizophrenic and their family. Being on the inside as a family member, it may often be very difficult to live with a loved one who has exhibited some of the symptoms that we identified earlier in this chapter. Studies relating to such difficulties suggest that relationships at home could be of crucial importance in influencing the frequency in which the individual may relapse. These realisations provide a rationale for the use of PSI. Read on to consider how studies have supported this view.

Expressed emotion within the family

A reader in sociology at the University of London, George Brown, together with two psychiatrists, undertook research which assessed the adjustment to the community of discharged mental patients. The initial study (Brown *et al.*, 1958) reviewed how patients coped after being discharged to live either with families or in lodging accommodation. They found that patients with schizophrenia were more likely to relapse if they returned to parents or spouses than if they went to live in lodgings or with brothers and sisters. This appeared a strange finding as they had expected that patients would receive more support from their families and hence would relapse less frequently.

In order to investigate the dynamics of home relationships and their impact upon the patient, Brown and his colleagues (1962) developed a structured interview schedule, **the Camberwell Family Interview (CFI)**, which would assess those households where patients were having problems and were relapsing as a result. The CFI was used with families to assess events and activities in the three months prior to the patient being admitted. The interview looked at attitudes and feelings toward the patient, as well as contact time and how family members carried out routine household tasks. The interviewers made a careful note of the amount of warmth, hostility and emotional over-involvement of family members toward the patient, and counted the frequency of positive or critical remarks made by the family about the patient (Brooker, 1990*b*). **They found that hostility, criticism or emotional over-involvement demonstrated by the family was closely correlated with relapse**.

These behaviours were defined in the following ways.

- **Hostility** is described as negative comments directly about the person, rather than their behaviour. An example might be: 'You never get out of bed. You're just a lazy good-for-nothing and will never be of any use to anybody.'

- **Criticism** is described as negative comments about the behaviour of the patient, an example being: 'I'm sick and tired of you leaving your dirty dishes in the sink. Will you get them washed for once.'

- **Emotional over-involvement** is described as the family member interfering or becoming so inseparable from the patient that they make

---

Understanding the client group and family needs **65**

decisions for them, control them and undertake their household tasks for them. An example of this behaviour might consist of giving up work or their free time to look after the patient, or continually speaking and acting on the patient's behalf. Family members may also become overtly over-emotional or greatly exaggerate the patient's situation, and be unable to separate their own feelings from those of the patient.

 Activity 2.15

Consider your responses to Activity 2.14 in relation to Robert.

- Is there any risk of you treating Robert in a critical, hostile or emotionally over-involved way?

- If so, what might be the underlying reasons for this?

Feedback to Activity 2.15

If you recognised that you were likely to be hostile, critical or over-involved then it may be an understandable reaction and you may have identified many reasons to approach Robert in such a way. We will move on now to further explore the impact of such approaches on the well-being of the patient.

The three behaviours of hostility, criticism and emotional over-involvement are described together as 'expressed emotion' (EE). If shown to be high in families, EE is significantly associated with relapse.

Further studies by Brown *et al.* (1972) revealed that the relapse rate nine months after discharge was 58% in patients experiencing high levels of EE within their home environment. This compares with a much lower relapse rate of 16% for those patients who were not faced with high EE at home. This was an important finding in that it clearly indicated situations that were making relapse far more frequent. Further research was needed in order to see if these significant results would be replicated.

The problem with the Camberwell Family Interview, however, was that it could take up to five hours to complete (Brooker, 1990*b*) and required lengthy training of interviewers. Vaughan and Leff (1976*a,b*) shortened the interview and used this to again follow the course of 43 discharged patients with a diagnosis of schizophrenia. Their results were combined with Brown's original data and again significant findings were noted.

However, their results found that other factors, apart from expressed emotion, were linked to relapse. Such factors were whether or not the patient was taking prescribed medication, and how much face-to-face time the patient actually spent with family members. Barrowclough and Tarrier (1984) found that:

- a low contact (less than 35 hours per week) and regular medication greatly reduced relapse in the high EE group (15%)

- a high contact and no medication resulted in a very high relapse rate (92%) (Figure 2.4).

This makes a great deal of sense. Even if there are high levels of EE then those patients who manage to minimise contact and gain benefits from medication can reduce its impact.

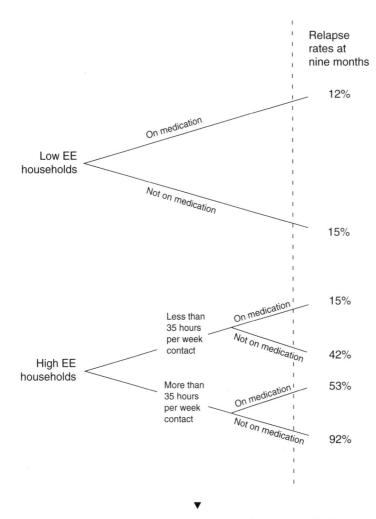

Figure 2.4 Differential relapse rates between high and low EE households (adapted from Brooker, 1990b).

THE STRESS-VULNERABILITY MODEL IN RELATION TO SCHIZOPHRENIA

Early research demonstrated that hostility, criticism and emotional over-involvement has a dramatic effect on the course of schizophrenia. These factors also appeared to be mediated by medication and face-to-face contact time. At the time that these studies were completed it was suggested by some clinicians that perhaps it was this sort of family interaction which actually resulted in the illness itself – that families caused schizophrenia! This led to some families being blamed for their relative's condition, and theories which attempted to explain that certain types of interaction between family members led to the development of schizophrenia. This is now known not to be the case, as the same communication and interaction problems are found within families caring for relatives with other physical conditions such as dementia or physical handicap.

A widely accepted theory, which has gained credence following this early research and subsequent intervention studies, is the '**stress-vulnerability model of schizophrenia**' (Zubin and Spring, 1977). Symptoms appear when a specific level of stress is reached. Patients who are living in family or other environments where levels of EE and tension are high will experience greater stress than patients living in environments where EE and tension are low. This is strongly supported by the EE studies referred to earlier, but is also supported by other research into the associations between stress and mental disorder. Cohen and Wills (1985) demonstrate that a supportive network enhances mental health by providing a **stress-mediating** or a **stress-buffering** role. Stress mediating occurs because the network provides regular positive experiences, a sense of stability and integration into a social role. Psychologically, the person receives social interaction and status support, which adds to the person's overall well-being. Stress buffering occurs when the person's network intervenes, either at the point when stress is first perceived, or in helping the person adapt to that stress. One of the most supportive aspects is the way in which the person is treated as an individual, in whom others are interested (Caplan 1974). Greenblatt *et al.* (1982) discuss research which demonstrates that strengthening and restructuring the support network of the mentally ill can enhance the course and outcome of treatment.

The stress-vulnerability model also suggests that individuals who develop schizophrenia have an enduring vulnerability trait or low stress tolerance, which is determined by genetic factors. Evidence suggests that certain biological factors, including arousal systems and information-processing systems in the brain, are dysfunctional in individuals who develop schizophrenia. It is this biological vulnerability together with a stressful environment that triggers schizophrenic symptoms. A possible representation of this model is shown in Figure 2.5.

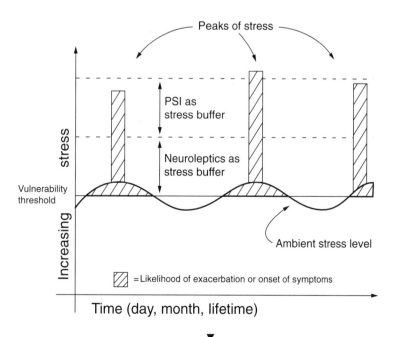

Figure 2.5 The stress-vulnerability model (adapted from Falloon *et al.*, 1984).

The continuous line in the graph represents environmental stress as it fluctuates up and down depending on the individual concerned. The blocks along this line represent sudden life-event stressors, such as sudden loss. The model postulates that when stress, either life event or environmental, passes the stress threshold then symptoms will occur. For individuals with an inherited vulnerability this threshold will be quite low. The graph also shows the effects of medication and learning effective coping strategies, both of which will raise the threshold so that the individual can cope with more stress, and hence experience symptoms less often. It is clear that if patients and their families can identify stress within the environment and reduce it, then the chances of relapse will be greatly diminished.

It is this model of schizophrenia and the body of early research which has provided a powerful rationale for attempting to intervene with families and schizophrenia sufferers. A series of family intervention studies have been implemented and evaluated which have aimed to alter high EE environments and enable patients and families to cope more effectively with stress. Various packages of care have been used which are now known as psychosocial interventions.

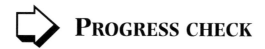 **PROGRESS CHECK**

In this chapter we have covered a great deal of ground, some or all of which may be new to you. We have considered the nature of schizophrenia – its symptoms, treatments and effects on the individual sufferer and family.

Before progressing to the next chapter you are invited to check your progress and ensure that you understand the material covered so far by answering the following questions. Check your answers against those given in Appendix 1.

1 List and give examples of the main types of problems associated with schizophrenia. One problem is given to start you off.

Disorders in thinking

2 Distinguish between positive and negative symptoms and give examples
   of each.

3 Describe the potential impact that a schizophrenia diagnosis could have
   on a family.

4 Identify the treatment approaches used for the care of schizophrenia.
  Discuss the aims of each approach.

5 List three changes in behaviour which may suggest relapse.

6 Identify three forms of early intervention which may prevent full relapse.

7 Describe the role of the Case Manager.

CHAPTER 3

The application of psychosocial interventions in practice

In Chapters 1 and 2 we considered the intervention needs of patients suffering from severe and enduring mental health problems. We identified therapies available and discussed general principles of care.

This chapter looks at PSI applied within the context of community care and as a potential approach for members of the primary healthcare team. We provide research evidence which supports the use of PSI and consider some ways in which PSI packages have been used and evaluated in practice.

Section 1 – The effects of working with families

So far we have looked at the nature of schizophrenia, the benefits of medication and the importance of low stress and low expressed emotion within home environments. In the last section we identified that schizophrenics may be particularly vulnerable to stress, and that the condition itself may bring stress into the family which is converted into high-expressed emotion. Within this section we will consider the impact of working with families to reduce stress by identifying and meeting the family's needs in relation to living with and caring for their loved one.

THE FAMILY INTERVENTION STUDIES

The following studies give some indication of the usefulness of PSI. The studies used a variety of methods to analyse the potency of the various single and combinations of interventions, and used relapse rates as indicators of effectiveness. When looking for some justification for using PSI, or encouraging others to consider their use, you may find it useful to refer to one or more of these studies.

Goldstein *et al.* (1978)

Goldstein *et al.* focused on a brief intervention aimed at developing crisis management within the family. A series of six sessions were designed to help the family plan how to avoid or cope with stressors which were influential in precipitating relapse in the patient. These six sessions were planned for patients immediately following discharge.

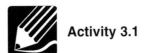 **Activity 3.1**

In Goldstein's study, a four-group design was used with 104 patients assigned randomly to one of the four groups:

1 intervention plus high dosage

2 intervention plus low dosage

3 high dosage only

4 low dosage only.

Consider these groups. What results would you expect in terms of relapse rates?

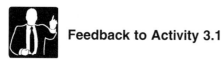 **Feedback to Activity 3.1**

The results demonstrated that the intervention plus high dosage group showed the lowest relapse rate (0%) at six-week and six-month follow-up, while the low dosage only group had the highest relapse rate (48%).

The researchers conclude that trends in the data strongly support the combined effects of an adequate dosage of neuroleptics and crisis-orientated family therapy in reducing relapse. Because it was so brief, being undertaken in six weeks, it is difficult to be certain that the intervention was the most important element of the research: after the six-week controlled period patients were treated in diverse ways. This makes it difficult to draw any conclusions from the six-month follow-up (Barrowclough and Tarnier, 1984).

Leff *et al.* (1982)

Leff and his colleagues developed a package of social interventions in their controlled trial. The package, which was tailored to each individual family, consisted of a four-session educational programme which:

• provided relatives with information regarding schizophrenia and its management

• set up a relatives group which was to enable support and a forum for learning more effective coping strategies

• provided individual family sessions which ranged from dynamic analysis to behavioural interventions.

Twenty-four families were randomly allocated to one of two treatment approaches which were either the social intervention package or routine out-patient care. All patients were receiving neuroleptic medication. The results demonstrated that 50% of the control group relapsed over nine months while only 9% relapsed in the intervention group. These figures suggest that the package was effective in reducing EE of the relatives and/or face-to-face contact time. In fact EE changed in both groups as did contact time, and more importantly it is not clear which elements of the package were effective.

Hogarty *et al.* (1986)

Hogarty *et al.* randomly allocated 103 patients to a four-group, two-year aftercare study in Pittsburgh, USA. The four groups comprised:

• family treatment and medication

• social skills training and medication

• combination of family interventions, social skills training and medication

• medication only.

The family treatment consisted of providing education and discussion of coping strategies in the management of schizophrenia. Its aim was to enable the family to attribute the patient's behaviour to illness rather than to him/herself, in order to reduce associated hostility and criticism. The social skills training consisted of behavioural techniques focused upon what was happening within the family.

In this study there were no relapses in the group receiving family interventions, social skills training and drug maintenance, while 41% of patients relapsed out of those receiving medication only. In discussion, they emphasise that these rates relate to a delay in relapse rather than prevention, and that at two-year follow-up 'relapse continues to rise in all experimental conditions'. This indicates that psychosocial interventions are effective, but that they need to be continued for long periods if relapse is to be prevented.

Falloon *et al.* (1985)

Falloon *et al.* randomly allocated 36 patients to either a family focused programme or an individual programme. The family programme consisted of behaviourally orientated problem-solving training which aimed to develop the families' skills in coping. Two sessions were devoted to education about schizophrenia with communication training given if needed. The individual programme again focused on problem solving and enhancing the patients' social functioning. Each programme consisted of 25 one-hour sessions.

After nine months a range of measures were used to demonstrate changes in the subjects. In terms of relapse, 6% in the family group compared favourably with 44% in the individual group. At two-year follow-up, 83% of the family group had not experienced a substantial exacerbation of schizophrenia, compared with only 17% in the individual group, thus confirming the efficacy of family-based management programmes over individual-orientated therapy in the community management of schizophrenia.

Tarrier *et al.* (1988)

Tarrier *et al.* used quite a complex design in order to differentiate between treatment conditions. They randomly allocated 64 high EE families to one of four groups:

- behavioural enactive (use of role play for problem solving)

- behavioural symbolic (use of verbal approaches such as teaching and discussion)

- education only

- routine treatment.

They also allocated 19 low EE families to either education only or routine treatment. The behavioural intervention consisted of two educational sessions, three stress management sessions and eight goal-setting sessions. They were taught using either symbolic methods of teaching, i.e. discussion and instruction, or enactive methods, i.e. role playing. The aims of the intervention were to reduce EE and raise the patients' level of functioning.

Results indicated that both behavioural interventions reduced relapse and changed relatives' EE status from high to low. They also showed that education alone did not reduce relapse in the high EE relatives group.

Barrowclough and Tarrier (1984)

Barrowclough and Tarrier discuss some of the issues raised by the research which focuses upon expressed emotion. They argue that other family interactions besides criticism, hostility and emotional over-involvement lead to stress within the family. They highlight Falloon *et al.*'s (1985) wider stress management approach to family intervention which is not limited to just the high EE families. They also argue for more research which will pinpoint the effects of each element of these psychosocial packages, suggesting that single-case experimental design might be a fruitful way forward.

Brooker and Butterworth (1991)

Brooker and Butterworth also raise the issue that much of this innovation has remained very much within the domain of researchers and not been taken up by the majority of clinicians, particularly nurses. They call for more effective and evaluated training of nurses in order to facilitate the results of these research studies into widespread clinical practice.

These studies show that psychosocial interventions are effective in reducing the chances of relapse within the first nine months following discharge (Lam, 1991). Further research needs to be undertaken into identifying the active interventions within these psychosocial programmes. This will mean broader assessment measures, including consumer questionnaires and the views of therapists and patients alike.

In summary, after 30 years of study it is clear that psychosocial interventions with patients and their families are beneficial in the management of schizophrenia (Hogarty *et al.*, 1986). These benefits are becoming increasingly validated with ever more specific research, to the point now that professionals are being urged to implement these programmes in everyday clinical practice. Nurses should be reviewing their current practice and adapting this body of research to their clinical settings.

Section 2 – Family work: the package

Although each intervention study used a slightly different clinical programme, there are certain common elements which can be drawn together into a 'package' which has been clearly demonstrated as being effective and evidence based.

Briefly, this programme of family intervention in the management of schizophrenia includes:

- **psychoeducation sessions** in which education is provided about schizophrenia – possible causes, symptoms, treatments and outcome – an emphasis being placed on the effects of stress within the family and how this can make symptoms worse

- **behavioural family work sessions** in which coping strategies are assessed, discussed and practical behavioural approaches used to improve coping skills. This work will involve **specific communication training and structured problem solving**.

In addition to the above specific interventions it is recognised that, to be effective, the delivery of psychosocial interventions needs to be within a context of multidisciplinary **case management** (see Chapter 2, Section 4), and care must be provided in a structured way, with clear goal setting and outcome measurements being evaluated regularly. This structured care should include accurate assessment of the needs of both patient and their family members, as well as identifying strengths. Each of these aspects of care delivery is outlined below.

PSYCHOEDUCATION

Psychoeducation is a common element in all of the family intervention studies previously discussed. The premise that education would be beneficial is mainly due to the idea that criticism and hostility occur as a result of feeling bewildered, frustrated or upset by the actions or inaction of the patient, including perhaps blaming them for their behaviour, which is in fact caused by their illness. Enabling the family to understand why the patient is behaving the way they are reduces the level of frustration felt, and leads to greater empathy rather than criticism. For this reason, educational programmes have tended to include information on symptoms, aetiology, medication, prognosis, and care and management. Some programmes are delivered on an individual family basis, others on a group basis. Programmes have also used different methods of delivery with varying lengths of sessions and frequency. An example of a psychoeducation programme is included in Appendix 2. This provides a working schedule of activities which are spread over four sessions.

A multifamily group was the basis for one programme in which nine sessions were delivered to three patients and their relatives (Liberman *et al.*, 1984). Anderson *et al.* (1980) also used groups of families together for an educational workshop spread over one day. They insist that feelings of isolation are reduced with a group format which increases interaction, support and allows for comparison with others. Miller (1989) offers a

---

psychoeducational approach to groups of patients using weekly sessions. He then has monthly sessions which include the patients' relatives or significant others. Further studies utilised the group concept in order to implement psychosocial programmes; all had similar formats and aimed to improve relatives' knowledge and coping strategies (Zelitch, 1980; Kyle and Taylor, 1983; Flannery and Link, 1986; Reid et al., 1993). Most also recognised the advantages of group work in providing peer support and a learning environment that allowed for the sharing of experiences and empathic understanding, and that:

> '...learning from peers meant getting information in an understandable form'. (Hatfield, 1990)

Many studies have also demonstrated the advantages of individual family work, either with or without the patient (Leff et al., 1982; McGill et al., 1983; Falloon et al., 1985; Greenberg et al., 1988; Tarrier et al., 1988). These studies implement a psychosocial programme for single families either in their home or within hospitals, and most wait until the patient is stabilised on medication before including them in family sessions. Falloon (1986) criticises this approach. Although acknowledging that acutely ill patients who lack insight about their condition are poor candidates for education, he nonetheless feels it is wrong to exclude the patient. By involving the patient from the start as as 'expert', their status within the family increases dramatically.

Most of the studies use a similar content in nearly all of their programmes, however, with all demonstrating some assessment and enhancement of coping skills to reduce stress. Some programmes also go on to include specific communication skills training and problem-solving training (Falloon et al., 1985), and cognitive-behavioural interventions with patients (Birchwood and Shepherd, 1992).

One programme has been developed and used by one of the contributors to this book (McCann and Clancy, 1996) for circumstances where a number of relatives may attend a central location for group sessions. The programme content is reproduced opposite, being more or less typical of the ground covered within common approaches to psychoeducation. The programme consisted of four two-hour sessions, and could be facilitated at weekends or evenings in order to engage relatives who might have difficulty attending at other times. Video, audio and written materials were used throughout the programme.

Numerous professionally produced audio-visual aids are available – these can be purchased or borrowed from public libraries; some have been put together and are distributed free of charge by the representatives of pharmaceutical firms. Similarly, there is a diversity of booklets and pamphlets written for relatives by a number of sources. Amongst the best of these are the series of booklets written by Birchwood and Smith (1991), which are available in a number of translated versions for various ethnic groups.

Structured Psychoeducation Programme

Session One

The aim of this session is to introduce the programme to relatives in detail; to discuss the needs of relatives in relation to both professional services and their relatives; and to raise awareness about schizophrenia from a sufferer's and relative's perspective.

- Introductions to group participants.

- Outline of four-session programme and format.

- Discussion: the needs of families and friends when not kept informed; the professional response and current research into schizophrenia and network support.

- Video: brief clip from tape which deals with the question 'what is schizophrenia?'

- Discussion: what is schizophrenia? Brainstorm what it means to group participants.

- Summary.

- Assignment. Each group participant to read booklets dealing with the issues 'What is schizophrenia?' and 'Help with schizophrenia'.

Session Two

The main aims of this session are to focus on the causes of schizophrenia that the relatives/friends are familiar with and to introduce the stress-vulnerability model of schizophrenia.

- Review assignment.

- Audio tape and discussion. Listen to the audio tape (dealing with the impact of schizophrenia on relatives and friends; stigma; confusion; worries about guilt/causes; grief and loss).

- Discussion: what are the relatives' perceptions of the causes of schizophrenia?

- Introduce the concept of the stress-vulnerability model of schizophrenia, based on what is known about causes.

- Assignment: relatives to find out the symptoms their family member is currently experiencing, or used to experience. Also the names and contact numbers of their family member's care team.

Continued

Continued

Session Three

The main aim of this session is to discuss in detail the symptoms of schizophrenia that relatives are familiar with; to introduce the concept of positive and negative symptoms; and to begin to understand coping strategies.

- Review assignment.

- Video 'Understanding Schizophrenia'.

- Brainstorm the symptoms relatives are familiar with (positive and negative). Introduce the concept of positive and negative symptoms. What control do patients have over their experiences? What makes symptoms easier or harder to cope with?

- Discussion: of the past problems relating to their family member's schizophrenia; how they coped with their family member; what they said or did to handle those situations.

Session Four

The main aim of this session is to discuss coping and handling situations that arise from having a relative/friend with schizophrenia.

- Discussion.

- General discussion about coping with symptoms. What makes them worse? What makes them better?

Key facts: – It's natural to feel angry and frustrated when somebody in the home is suffering from symptoms.

- Stress within the household should be kept to a minimum (hostility, criticism, over-involvement).

- It's important that you take care of yourself and continue to live a full life.

- When problems arise it helps to solve them together in a structured way.

- It is important to know where to go for help and to be aware of what services exist *before* you need them.

- Try to maintain contact with friends, relatives and colleagues.

- Specific strategies for specific symptoms can be adopted following assessment of problems. Help with this can be sought from the primary nurse, the care team or rehab staff.

- Remember that the problem behaviours are caused by schizophrenia and not by the individual.

Smith and Birchwood (1987) note that education is not purely an academic exercise to increase knowledge, but that it has many other non-specific effects. One they note is the relatives' perception of 'being' or 'feeling' more knowledgeable, which in itself raises confidence and control over the situation. They go on to say that, overall, an educational programme can enable and empower relatives to become more involved in further work.

Brooker (1990a) summarises many other needs relatives have, many of which can be met by education. Carers feel anxious trying to cope with bizarre symptoms, their social life is often greatly reduced, they feel depressed because nothing they do seems to help, and they feel guilty because professionals often lead them to suspect that they are to blame. Often they experience grief for the 'normal' person they have now lost. A recognition of these burdens and a concern for the relatives' needs should be an integral part of any educational approach (Berkowitz, 1984). McGill et al. (1983) stated that following their educational programme, relatives' confusion, uncertainty and unrealistic expectations, which gave rise to a great deal of distress, were alleviated. Family members tended to be less critical and more supportive, and an increased understanding of the role of medication was found.

The content of educational programmes does not seem to matter so much as how it is delivered. In fact, Smith and Birchwood (1987) state that '... content is irrelevant as a medium of change'.

It appears to be the delivery of the education and its utility to the families which are the critical factors (Barrowclough et al., 1987). Brooker et al. (1992) distinguish between two main methods of education: the deficit model and the interactive model. They argue that giving 'blanket information' to relatives in a rather didactic way is not only patronising but highly uneconomic. The interactive model first assesses what the relatives already believe and attempts to use that knowledge in as positive a way as possible, whilst at the same time introducing other ideas. Tarrier and Barrowclough (1986) outline six guidelines concerning the delivery of education about schizophrenia. The first appears the most important: 'There is a need to assess and take into account both patients' and relatives' perceptions of the illness ... information is not given in a vacuum.'

It is the interactive process of giving and receiving information that generates the other benefits of psychoeducation described earlier – the reduced sense of burden, the optimism, reduced feeling of distress and a sense of control over the situation.

Tarrier et al. (1988) reported, however, in their controlled trial that an educational component by itself did not alter the EE of relatives from high to low, or have a corresponding impact on relapse rates. Two other controlled trials involving an educational component in the intervention (Leff et al., 1982; Falloon et al., 1985) demonstrated a reduced relapse rate, but failed to be explicit about the effect the educational component actually had (Barrowclough and Tarrier, 1992).

Berkowitz (1984) provides a fuller description and interpretation of the concept of EE as it applied to the study by Leff et al. (1982). She presents some interesting insights into the measurement, particularly of low EE, stating that low EE has no specific definition except in terms of an absence of characteristics. Low EE is seen as being neutral or passive whereas in fact low EE relatives play an active role in reducing arousal within the patient. She criticises the grouping of all high EE relatives together as there are marked differences in their interactive styles, particularly between critical and over-involved relatives. She also deliberates about the role education plays in the therapeutic process and recognises its positive and negative elements, for example the disadvantages of labelling the patient as ill as well as, in contrast, the advantages of removing guilt about the family as the cause. She strikes a balance in recognising that education is a way of helping the relatives become more sympathetic and sensitive to their role in the patient's condition. Her paper neatly raises our understanding of how interventions are based upon assessed needs.

It is clear that education about schizophrenia for relatives has many varied and complex benefits, quite apart from the acquisition of knowledge. Therefore a programme would be limited if it sought only to alter EE status of relatives – many other aims of a psychosocial package need to be considered.

Communication skills training

Following on from the educational programme, during which it is emphasised that coping with someone who has schizophrenia can be difficult and emotionally draining, it is then acknowledged that how the patient and family interact can be crucial in terms of raising or lowering stress levels. Discussions about how the patient and family cope with schizophrenia will have identified areas of communication which may not be of benefit in ensuring that stress remains low. It is therefore essential to enlist the patient and family's support in improving the way they interact in order to reduce the chances of a relapse occuring.

Falloon *et al.* (1993) use a behavioural model to train families how to use a range of communication skills which will help them solve problems and cope more effectively with stress. They recognise four essential communication skills which are particularly helpful in reducing stress:

- expressing positive feelings

- making a positive request

- expressing unpleasant feelings

- attentive listening.

Their programme ensures that each family member is able to use these skills effectively in order to reduce the risks of relapse. The method used for training families to use these skills follows several key steps.

1 **Agreeing a rationale** with the family for learning a communication skill is the first step. This should be straightforward and focused on why it is important to learn the particular skill. Using expressing positive feelings as an example, the agreed rationale might include: the importance of giving people encouragement, the need to focus on the strengths rather than the weaknesses of others and feeling appreciated and valued. Each family member would need to agree to work on this skill before the next step.

2 **Role playing the skill** allows the family to describe and act out the present communication skill currently used by family members. The family would be encouraged to elicit an example of how they express positive feelings to one another, e.g. how one family member appreciates the patient doing an everyday household task.

3 **Constructive feedback** is then provided to the family member demonstrating the skill, such as eye contact, tone of voice, stating clearly what was appreciated and describing how it made them feel. Positive feedback is provided first, followed by suggestions of how they might have demonstrated the skill more effectively. It is at this point that family members often realise how difficult it is to communicate effectively, and how everyone can learn to enhance their communication skills.

4 **Repeated practice** of the skill is then continued until it is performed competently.

All of the above steps are repeated with each of the four key skills, until each skill can be demonstrated by each family member. The whole aim of this very structured training method is that behaviours learned within the family sessions are then transferred into everyday interactions. This is further reinforced using homework assignments which are completed by the family between sessions.

PROBLEM-SOLVING TRAINING

Enabling the family members to communicate effectively with one another will allow effective problem solving to be undertaken, and the development of enhanced coping strategies. In order to aid this process, specific training in problem-solving skills is provided in the Falloon *et al.* (1993) programme. Here, the emphasis is on the family learning to be precise in establishing what the problem is, agreeing the problem with all family members and then using a structured approach to generate a plan to cope with the problem more effectively.

Falloon *et al.* (1993) used a six-step method for solving problems and asks one family member to write down the discussion on problem-solving worksheets:

1 **Pinpoint the problem** as precisely as possible. This may take some time but it is important to agree what the problem is before attempting to deal with it. Often when discussing the problem it becomes clear that there are really several problems which impinge on each other. It is necessary to try and separate out which is the key issue and focus just on this. Similarly, different family members may have a variety of views on the actual nature of the problem.

2 **List all possible solutions** to the problem selected. It is important just to brainstorm ideas at this stage, whether appropriate or not, and to try and get each family member to generate at least one solution.

3 **Weigh up each possible solution** by discussing briefly the advantages and disadvantages of each one.

---

4 **Choose the best solution** or at least the one that can be applied within available resources and which will solve at least part of the problem. Debate about which is the best solution is sometimes needed, during which good communication skills should be promoted.

5 **Plan how to carry out the best solution** in sufficient detail so that each family member is clear about what is expected, who is going to do what, when and how. At this stage it is worth attempting to identify what problems may be encountered in carrying out the plan, and when the plan will be reviewed.

6 **Review the plan**, noting whether it has worked and what has been achieved. If the plan needs modifying this should be done with everyone's agreement. If the solution chosen has not worked, another solution may be selected and again another plan implemented.

Family members are encouraged to discuss problems as a group in order to generate as many solutions and perspectives as possible, and all share in the plan to solve the problem. This emphasises that problems affect everyone within a family and are not solely the responsibility of one person, and that the family can solve problems in a structured way without the need for professional intervention.

This structured, step-by-step method can also be used to consider either individual or family goals, and it is this emphasis on promoting strengths which is advocated by Barrowclough and Tarrier (1992). Their methods take a constructionist approach to presenting problems by asking the question 'If the patient didn't have the problem, what would they be doing?' This is opposite to the problem-focused method which says 'How can we reduce or eliminate this behaviour?'

Again they use a very structured cognitive-behavioural approach, but reframe problems into needs and plans into goals to be achieved. For example, the problem may be that the patient spends too long lying around doing nothing. This problem would be translated into the patient needing to spend more time doing activities. A list of patient and family strengths, interests and resources would be made, and a plan drawn up providing step-by-step achieveable goals. Again, time would be set aside by the family to discuss and review the progress of the plan in achieving the goal.

Section 3 – Assessing need

Assessing patients and their care, evaluating outcomes and reviewing services are key themes in the organisation of care for any client group, but with clients whose needs are complex, and for whom support and treatment may be provided by a diversity of disciplines, they are essential. Assessments and evaluations of outcome have been rigorously applied in most studies which have implemented psychosocial interventions. This has not only been because of the need to evaluate the clinical programmes themselves, but, more importantly, it is an integral part of the cognitive-behavioural model itself. This emphasises the need for accurate and detailed assessments of need in order to plan and set realistic targets. These targets are set in collaboration with the patient and their family, and outcomes measured and discussed as part of the therapeutic process.

For these reasons most studies have used a range of assessments besides relapse rate as a means of identifying the therapeutic benefits of their psychosocial programmes. Table 3.1 highlights several studies and the range of assessment tools they used.

Assessments used can be grouped under those that assess the needs of patients or those that assess the needs of their families.

For patients, the main outcome measure is that which assesses mental state. This may consist of a structured assessment interview such as the Present State Examination (Wing *et al.*, 1974) or the Manchester Scale (Krawiecka *et al.*, 1977). These assess items such as anxiety, depression, psychotic symptoms or behavioural problems. Other mental state assessments may look at symptoms in more detail such as depression (Beck *et al.*, 1979) or hallucinations or delusions. Others may attempt to identify early warning signs that symptoms are returning or getting worse (Birchwood *et al.*, 1989), or to measure social functioning (Birchwood *et al.*, 1990) or the amount of insight the patient has into their own problems.

Family assessments consist mainly of two assessment areas. The first is knowledge about schizophrenia (Barrowclough and Tarrier, 1992) which each family member holds, and is usually completed before and following an educational programme. The second is how family members interact with the patient, what their concerns are and how they cope with problem behaviours (Barrowclough and Tarrier, 1992). Other assessments have been used which aim to assess the amount of distress the family members are experiencing with regard to the patient's problems.

Table 3.1: Assessment tools utilised in intervention studies

Study	Measures
Leff *et al.* (1982)	• Camberwell Family Interview • Present State Examination
McGill *et al.* (1983)	• Knowledge Questionnaire
Liberman *et al.* (1984)	• Camberwell Family Interview • Knowledge Questionnaire • Family Conflict Inventory • Present State Examination • Psychiatric Assessment Scale • Relapse Rate • Consumer Satisfaction Scale
Falloon *et al.* (1984)	• Brief Psychiatric Rating Scale • Relapse Rate • Present State Examination • Hopkins Symptom Check-list
Doane *et al.* (1986)	• Affective Style Measure • Problem-solving Style • Relapse Rate
Hogarty *et al.* (1986)	• Camberwell Family Interview • Relapse Rate
Barrowclough *et al.* (1987)	• Camberwell Family Interview • Knowledge About Schizophrenia Interview

Smith and Birchwood (1987)	• Assessment Questionnaire to measure:
	  – Knowledge (beliefs, worry, disturbance)
	  – Symptom Rating Test
	  – Family Distress Scale

Tarrier *et al.* (1988)	• Camberwell Family Interview • Present State Examination • Social Functioning Scale • General Health Questionnaire • Symptom Rating Test • Family Questionnaire
Reid *et al.* (1993)	• Symptom Rating Test • Family Distress Scale • Severity of Patient Disturbance • Knowledge About Schizophrenia Interview

Section 4 – Psychosocial interventions in primary care

MENTAL HEALTH PROBLEMS IN PRIMARY CARE

Britain has one of the best primary care services in the world with 98% of the population being registered with a general practitioner (GP). The average GP list has approximately 2010 patients.

In any one year 60% of those patients registered will consult their GP, with between one-fifth to one-quarter having a mental health problem either as a sole or major component of their presentation (Strathdee *et al.*, 1996). The majority of presenting mental health problems in primary care fall into the 'less severe' areas, with about one-tenth having a chronic disorder; this being defined as continually present for one year or requiring prophylactic treatment. It is important to note that primary care has traditionally dealt with the bulk of mental health morbidity within its own team structures, with GPs referring only one in ten of their patients to specialist mental health services in secondary care.

In the recent past, liaison between primary and secondary care has taken place around groups of patients referred by GPs to consultant psychiatrists for domiciliary visits or out-patient assessments, involving links with large psychiatric hospitals or psychiatric units attached to district general hospitals. Referral practices for GPs vary considerably and the following features are common considerations for GP referral patterns to secondary care:

- male

- young

- not responding to GP treatment

- requests made by relatives

- suicidal

- have presenting behavioural problems in the community.

The importance of shared care development was recognised by the Royal Colleges of Psychiatrists and General Practitioners and details were published in their joint report of 1993. This aimed to produce a consensus acknowledging the problems created by the rapid expansion of care in the community developments. The report recognised that both psychiatry and general practice share an interest in treating the whole patient, and that developments in community psychiatry and primary care had increasingly blurred boundaries between GPs and psychiatrists.

This report is summarised in the following key areas for development:

- **The alignment of catchment areas** – achieving co-terminous boundaries with other agencies will improve referral access and communications overall

- **consultant liaison links** – the report stressed the need for face-to-face contact; best assured by the consultant reviewing their patients in the GP's surgery

---

- **clinical responsibility** – patients seen at the GP's surgery should remain the responsibility of the GP in terms of regular prescribing and the routine review of physical and mental health. Clearly, the role of the consultant and community mental health team must be defined and agreed, particularly for those patients recently discharged from hospital and/or under the restrictions of the Mental Health Act

- **joint audit** – the need to monitor prescribing and admissions to hospital, setting up practice-based disease or case registers for assistance in the management of the severely mentally ill (SMI) at local practice levels

- **close integration of training** – over 40% of GP trainees are now receiving training in a psychiatric post. There remains the need for further collaboration and integration between local medical training programmes.

More than any other area of healthcare specialisms, psychiatry and general practice have developed new approaches to their work, the most important of these being working in teams. The government's programme of de-institutionalisation has placed an increased burden on GPs and primary care teams (Thornicroft and Bebbington, 1989). The steady reduction in hospital beds for people with mental health problems has futher compounded the difficulties for those working in the primary care setting. Those areas without adequate community provision of crisis care or respite facilities, or a well-developed and robust Care Programme Approach (CPA) supported with Care Management teams, have particular problems. Further to this, areas that are undertaking home-based treatments as an alternative to hospital admission have particular difficulty in developing new practice (Strathdee, 1992).

Jenkins (1992) explains that at its most fundamental the purpose of a health service is to achieve some overall health gain and improve the health of the nation. National strategy sets targets for mental health services to reduce ill health and death caused by severe mental illness. The management of existing illness is essential and it is important to slow down the rate of deterioration of incurable diseases and to minimise accompanying social disability, improving the individual and family's quality of life.

It is important to agree the division of clinical boundaries and responsibilities between primary care and community mental health teams to ensure continuity of care provision, considering the social care needs of patients in collaboration with social services departments and their Care Managers. Community mental health teams should develop agreements and protocols to communicate mechanisms for routine and emergency contact, with all concerned receiving a copy of the patient/client community care plan. These care plans are ideally agreed under the CPA, coordinated through a key worker in a collaborative approach, securing links and future development in the primary care setting.

The NHS Executive also recognises that the collaboration between mental health services, social services and general practice is an important part of the implementation of the CPA. The Priority and Planning Guidance 1997/98 reaffirms a commitment to ensuring CPA is fully implemented and audited.

Involvement of the primary care team with the care programme in their practice and locality has benefits for both general practitioners, their patients and carers, and it is a key area and the development responsibility of community mental health teams to build on this initiative.

Data collected from the 1960s to 1980s indicate that GPs were closely involved with the management of people with schizophrenia. Reports have consistently demonstrated that up to 25% of patients with schizophrenia in the community discharged from mental health facilities were managed only by their family doctor. GPs have borne a sizeable burden of the care in the community initiatives with patients suffering from long-term mental illness, sometimes without assistance from secondary care. There is an urgent need for more information on the management of patients with chronic schizophrenia in primary care, and the presumption that GPs only concern themselves with patients who present with anxiety and depression has been strongly challenged (King, 1992).

Liaison psychiatry, in which psychiatrists work directly within general practice settings, has been rapidly expanding in the UK. Protocols for mental health practice in the primary care setting require that methods of secondary prevention are developed. Liaison clinics have been increasing in number since the early 1970s, albeit in an *ad hoc* fashion. The advantage is ease of access to information and review for patients. The disadvantages crystallise around concerns that these clinics will be dominated by the more demanding 'worried well', at the cost of those patients with SMI. There is no obvious sign that this is the case and the CPA mechanisms should ensure this is an issue that is under regular review.

Community mental health nurses from secondary care multidisciplinary teams are ideally placed to facilitate shared care or liaison clinic developments in the primary care setting, as they are usually the main key workers under the CPA for those people with serious mental illness and have a good working knowledge of both secondary care systems and local community resources.

The development of a primary care-led NHS was heralded in 1996, switching the emphasis from secondary care provision. The White Paper *Primary Care: The Future – Choice and Opportunity*, published in October 1996, responded directly to calls for greater flexibility and set out proposals for legislation. The NHS and Primary Care Bill offers opportunities to improve services for the benefit of patients at a local level. It is envisaged that better team working between professionals will enable patients to receive a more integrated service at home. Patients in the inner cities will benefit from new initiatives, and elderly and mentally ill people will, for example, benefit from greater opportunities for primary care teams to include speicalist professionals and mental health staff. GP fundholding arrangements have been in place in most areas for some years, and the primary care initiative allows the opportunity for local needs-based services to develop.

Allocation of scarce resources will always be an issue. The challenge for mental health services is to develop their work for people with serious and enduring mental health problems, while supporting and assisting changes and new initiatives in the primary care team in the treatment of less severe mental health problems. The government has implemented policies and legislation that ensure that those people with SMI are focused upon by specialist mental health services. The major difficulty for the community mental health nurses (CMHN) and community mental health team (CMHT) is to maintain this focus and support GP and primary care team developments. Barker (1993) points out the danger of dismissing people as the 'worried well' because they are not suffering from psychosis, and that people with illnesses such as depression are often described as 'less seriously ill', but such a disorder can have devastating and long-standing effects for the individual and their family. Careful thought has to be given in making such statements since assumptions can be made about who is deserving of the services of mental health teams. Nevertheless, it is essential that services are prioritised and that this does not mean devoting all of the CMHT's attention on one particular group, nor should these teams expect to meet the mental health needs, in totality, for everyone who is referred. Priority setting is about altering the balance of existing resources and redeploying them for the maximum benefit of patient care.

Traditionally the SMI population have been cared for in the large psychiatric institutions and presented few problems for the GP and primary care team. There is now a need for secondary care services to support the GP and primary care team in becoming more proactive in the management of the range of presenting mental health problems. This will undoubtedly involve taking time to deal with those who present with minor mental health problems *and* continuing development work with the locally based SMI population using the CPA and psychosocial interventions.

The psychosocial approaches are best used in conjunction with CPA and Care Management arrangements. It is important to develop this structure and adapt some of these approaches to meet the needs of both SMI and less severe mental health problems through liaison with CMHTs in the primary care setting.

Gournay and Brooking (1994) reports that community mental health nurses are increasingly working in primary healthcare with non-psychotic patients, and supports developments that ensure people with SMI are focused upon. In this respect, it can be argued that patients with chronic schizophrenia are in danger of neglect, and that community mental health nurses should refocus their activity and education on appropriate skills acquisition and interventions of proven effectiveness, ensuring research-based practice (Gournay and Brooking, 1994). Lancashire and colleagues (1995) conclude that psychiatric nurses are ideally placed to deliver psychosocial interventions, and more widespread dissemination of these skills and approaches will enable them to fulfil more completely the expectations implicit in the recent Mental Health Nursing Review (1994), which highlights a shift towards collaboration between primary and secondary mental health nursing care.

Falloon *et al.* (1990) postulate that where close liaison with family practitioners is established, it may prove feasible to detect initial episodes of florid schizophrenia at a much earlier stage than usual, and to treat the disorder before the onset of serious social disability and handicap. Falloon (1992) points out the refinements over the past two decades in the long-term management of schizophrenia, reminding us that while the recovery rate remains around 20%, florid episodes and exacerbations of schizophrenia have been controlled more effectively to enable care in the community initiatives to develop. The use of low-dosage neuroleptic medication with the addition of a broad range of psychosocial interventions targeted at patients and families most at risk, supported by systematic case management, allows the care in the community initiative to move on.

As a starting point the CMHT could assist future developments in primary care by supporting initiatives similar to those outlined above which would modify and develop approaches to mental health assessment at practice level. This would need to be supported by alternative systems of prioritising mental health referral practices while maintaining the SMI focus within primary care.

EARLY DETECTION OF SERIOUS MENTAL HEALTH PROBLEMS

We considered relapse in some detail in Chapter 2. Here we consider a particular staged approach which is appropriate to primary healthcare. Falloon (1992) provides us with a useful two-stage approach to primary care and CMHT developments in early detection procedures for schizophrenia:

- **stage one** – training family practitioners to recognise prodromal signs for schizophrenia and without delay refer such people

- **stage two** – immediate specialised mental health assessment (within 24 hours):

    - **Early Signs Questionnaire** (Hertz and Melville, 1980) for the patient and the care giver. If this suggests a prodromal state then the **Present State Examination** (PSE) is completed by the mental health professional.

This service is offered together with the following check-list for GPs (Falloon, 1992) that outlines eight features that might indicate the early stage of an acute episode of schizophrenia, derived from the prodromal signs outline in DSM-111 (APA, 1980).

Prodromal symptoms of schizophrenia

Onset of one of the following without explanation:

- marked peculiar behaviour

- inappropriate or loss of affect

- vague, rambling speech

- marked poverty of speech and thought

- preoccupation with odd ideas

- ideas of reference

- depersonalisation or derealisation

- perceptual disturbances.

Early Intervention Programme

This includes the following:

- education about the nature of schizophrenia

- home-based stress management

- neuroleptic medication

- problem solving with families.

Close collaboration and support within the primary care setting together with an **assertive outreach model** of care provided by the community-based mental health service are essential components of this approach. This has led to improved case finding at a local level, but it is unlikely that all new cases will be found in the primary care setting.

Work to identify early signs or indication of SMI in the primary care setting has taken place with some success. Assisting GPs to look for early warning signs in their patients, with a view to monitoring and supporting those who may be developing serious mental health problems, is an important secondary prevention measure and forms the initial development of a psychosocial intervention approach in primary care. Together with the provision and assistance of new medication treatments, a team approach can lead to a more proactive way forward to assessment, treatment and management of first episodes of SMI in the primary care setting.

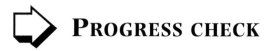 **PROGRESS CHECK**

1 Within Section 1 of this chapter we summarised a selection of research-based studies which looked at the usefulness of PSI for patients suffering from schizophrenia, and their families. Think back to those studies and, using evidence presented, write about 500 words to justify the use of PSI for the named client group.

Unlike progress checks in Chapters 1 and 2 there are no answers summarised in Appendix 1. You may like to complete questions 1 and 2 and share your responses with colleagues in order to gain their perspectives and to ellicit team discussion.

2 Listed below are three examples of interventions used within PSI:

• psychoeducation

• communication skills training

• structured problem solving.

Choose one example and answer the questions which follow.

a What are the aims of the chosen intervention?

b Describe the role of the therapist for the intervention.

c What participation is required of the patient?

d What participation is required of the patient's family?

CHAPTER 4
Development needs for primary healthcare teams

At this point you may be considering ways in which you, and your colleagues, may start to use PSI within your practice.

Within this chapter you will be given an opportunity to identify what issues need to be addressed in order to modify practice in line with the philosophy of PSI.

The material here will provide a summary to the earlier parts of the book. It will also enable you to envisage how you can enhance your practice for the benefit of clients with severe and enduring mental health problems.

Section 1 – Review of principles of care

When considering how best to meet the needs of clients with SMI within your care, the following aspects should be considered:

- challenging stigma
- supporting the carer
- collaboration with other service providers
- recognising vulnerability
- evaluation of input.

 Activity 4.1

Consider the above five aspects of care in turn and identify ways in which you would deal with each one within your practice.

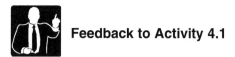 **Feedback to Activity 4.1**

You should now have some thoughts relating to dealing with stigma, supporting the carer, working with other agencies, recognising vulnerability and evaluating care. Your responses will relate to your own current practice situation.

Now read on to consider the author's advice relating to each aspect of care and use it to complement what you included.

CHALLENGING STIGMA

The challenge for primary care mental health teams is to maintain the focus of care for those people with SMI and develop new initiatives which support appropriate services for those who present with less serious mental health problems. The consequence of inadequately treated depression and anxiety in the primary care setting is often referral on to mental health services, bringing with it associated difficulties, for example sick role reinforcement, stigma and labelling for this group. The need to use prevention and health promotion for all people with mental health problems is an appropriate area to build and develop into the work of primary care mental health teams, with a view to the provision of greater access to appropriate helping services and agencies.

McKeown and Clancy (1995) suggest that nurses whose practice involves health promotion or the support of clients in the community should have particular interest in the mechanisms by which popular images of mental illness and media influences are generated and how these affect people's everyday lives. Hallam (1997) states that the general public are now familiar with psychiatric symptoms, diagnosis and side effects of medication in a way which would have been unthinkable in the days when people were cared for in large institutions. However, she goes on to say the greater exposure to the issues appears to have little effect in reducing stigma associated with mental illness and that negative attitudes have become increasingly entrenched.

The stigmatisation of mental illness increases stress and results in a reduction in quality of lives, adding to the social isolation that often goes in conjunction with having a serious mental illness. The development of mental health prevention and promotion work at primary care level can be an important contribution to dismantling such attitudes. This ought to include reflection upon one's own attitudes as a practitioner within the team, including awareness of gender and cultural issues.

CARER SUPPORT

Aside from the need for structured programmes of family therapy, there is a much more general need for the support of informal carers in the community. The shift towards community care by necessity places a burden upon families and other concerned individuals. The carers of any chronically ill persons will undoubtedly be in need of varying degrees of both emotional and practical support, some of which could be facilitated within GP practices. Perhaps the bringing together of families whose mutual commonalities revolve around the need for support *per se*, rather than involvement with any particular illness or condition, might be a means of dismantling stigma through the recognition of shared experiences in apparently dissimilar circumstances.

Other groups in the voluntary sector, such as MIND, the Hearing Voices network, or Making Space, may provide local support groups or resource centres. Similarly, there may be some statutory provision of this sort, provided by the local community mental health services for instance. If this is the case then it might be opportune for primary care staff to collate such information as location and dates of meetings within their resource directory.

It must also be recognised that the need for such support might also extend to the professional carers, charged with the responsibility of looking after this client group within the variety of community-based residential facilities.

SERVICE USER INVOLVEMENT

Models of collaborative and participatory care are becoming more and more appropriate within modern health services, not least because of a wider trend towards consumerism. In this context we can conceive of both the sufferers of severe and enduring problems and their families as having an interest in becoming involved in services. It is usually the case that when such people are asked what they want from services they ask for three things:

- better information

- more involvement

- emotional and practical support.

Greater involvement of patients and their families in exploring the complexities of their problems, history taking and the planning and delivery of care is essential if psychosocial interventions are to be effective.

ASSESSMENT OF RISK AND VULNERABILITY

It is important that primary care teams are both involved and supported in the assessment and management of risk and vulnerability in this client group. It is not uncommon, with hindsight, to be able to point out deficiencies in the management of risk and vulnerability in the community. A typical shortcoming is lack of appropriate liaison and exchange of information between interested professionals and agencies. Just as important has been the lack of involvement of families as valuable informants regarding deterioration in mental state and worries about possible consequences. It is essential that family members who seek help regarding concerns about suicide risk or potential for other harms, say violence, have their concerns taken seriously. This ought to involve specialist services as appropriate.

The consequences of suicide or violent incidents in the community are devastating for all involved – the victims, families and the professionals concerned. The minimisation of these risks is in everybody's interests, and is a priority area of current health policy. Of course, it is almost axiomatic that not all serious risk can be predicted. As such, primary care services may from time to time be necessarily involved in coping with the aftermath of awful and distressing events. This could range from providing bereavement support for the families of suicide victims, or caring for the victims of serious crime, and their families. It is important to remember here that the families of mentally disordered offenders in this context assume a status similar to that of victims, and will also require our support.

EVALUATION AND AUDIT

Any modification in the practice of healthcare or the implementation of new systems of working ought to be monitored and evaluated systematically. This might be as simple a task as auditing activity levels in relation to the provision of services for specific groups. More interesting is the evaluation of effectiveness of different means of delivering services. There are a variety of tools available for assessing patient-centred outcomes concerning the progress of symptoms and problems, general quality of life measures and satisfaction with specific services. Global assessments of need within practices, such as the Camberwell Assessment of Need, or outcomes, such as the HONOS – or Health of the Nation Outcome Scale, are available for use by the team.

Section 2 – What next? Personal action plan

Up to this point we hope that you have developed an interest in PSI and an appreciation of their value to your practice.

There are additional materials in Appendix 3 which relate to ways in which the effectiveness of the primary team may be enhanced and a 'tool kit' which acts as a resource for enhancing practice. Appendix 4 provides information about practitioner training in PSI.

You may wish to look at the additional materials and reflect for a while to decide on what, if anything, you wish to do now to incorporate your new learning into practice.

Action plan

Appendix one

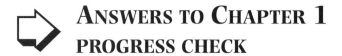

ANSWERS TO CHAPTER 1
PROGRESS CHECK

1 What are psychosocial interventions (PSI)?

Psychosocial interventions are any form of therapeutic interaction which has psychological and social dimensions. Within your experience you may have used, or heard of, such interventions in the care of the dying, within counselling situations, or for the care of the mentally ill.

2 What client groups in particular may benefit from the use of PSI, and why?

Though useful for a variety of client groups, PSI are particularly useful within mental healthcare and in the care of individuals with severe and enduring mental health problems, usually having a diagnosis of schizophrenia. In this context PSI are used as an approach to dealing with the diversity of problems such people may face. (These problems relate to actual symptoms as well as social and psychological problems which occur as a consequence of having been diagnosed schizophrenic.) They require more than just medication in order to help them and their families to live with optimum quality of life. PSI address social and psychological needs and aim to develop individual and family coping responses.

3 List three examples of PSI.

Your list may have included any of the following interventions:

- **anything that reduces stress or its impact** – either by modifying the social environment in some way, or by enhancing people's coping strategies. These interventions might include:

  - anxiety management sessions

  - taught relaxation techniques

  - distraction (like listening to music)

- **family therapy**, incorporating:

  - psychoeducation

  - communication skills training

  - problem-solving skills training

- **cognitive behavioural therapy** for psychotic symptoms

- **early warning signs monitoring**.

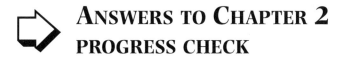

ANSWERS TO CHAPTER 2
PROGRESS CHECK

1 List and give examples of the main types of problems associated with schizophrenia.

There is a whole range of problems which an individual may experience if suffering from schizophrenia. You may have included some or all of the following:

- disorders in thinking

- hallucinations

- delusions

- negative symptoms

- depression

- anxiety

- suicidal ideas

- problematic drug use

- sleep disturbance

- effects on relationships

- sexual problems

- stigma.

Remember, an individual may not experience all of these problems but may present with groupings of them which may be unique to him/her. The label of schizophrenia may be based on a variety of problems presented.

2 Distinguish between positive and negative symptoms and give examples of each.

Positive symptoms, such as hallucinations, delusions and thought disorder, are additions to the person's life experience. You and I do not, if well, experience these symptoms because they are not present normally. Negative symptoms, however, are losses of life experiences which are present in everyone's daily life experiences. Examples of negative symptoms are loss of zest for life, loss of drive, apathy and difficulties in relating spontaneously to people. In health the person with schizophrenia would have been motivated, interested and able to form attachments to people, but schizophrenia takes these abilities away or diminishes them noticeably.

3 Describe the potential impact that a schizophrenia diagnosis could have on a family.

Using experience of clients, insights from your reflections during Activity 2.14 and from working through Chapter 2 you may have been able to describe the range of responses possible by family members. You may have identified feelings of shame, fear and bewilderment. You may have described ways in which family members attempt to cope by being over-protective or critical. The actual responses depend upon the existing family dynamics at the time, and the impact will vary. The impact may include loss of an income-earner, loss of a loving relationship and reduction in social enjoyment; it could take the form of being ashamed and wishing to stay hidden from neighbours. The responses to schizophrenia can be assessed in terms of expressed emotion where such behaviours as hostility, criticism and over-involvement can be considered in relation to the sufferer within the family.

4 Identify the treatment approaches used for the care of schizophrenia. Discuss the aims of each approach.

You should have identified two main types of treatment approaches. These are:

- **physical, in the form of medication** classed as neuroleptic or antipsychotic agents. These are used to control the symptoms, both positive and negative, which may be present. They may, through acting upon the neurotransmitters, dampen down positive symptoms and some may act incisively to cut through the negative symptoms and stimulate greater interactivity with the environment.

- **psychological interventions** which may take the form of behavioural techniques such as rewarding changes in behaviour, thought management interventions such as thought stopping to counteract hallucinations, reality testing to challenge delusions, social skills training to improve social interaction and functioning, and psychosocial interventions which aim to reeducate and support individuals and their families in coping with the problems presented in a constructive way.

5 List three changes in behaviour which may suggest relapse.

Individuals may present with behaviours that are peculiar to them and which may, through the experienced and informed eye of the carer, be reliable signs of deterioration in their mental health. You may have listed any or all of the following examples:

- spending more time alone in bedroom

- becoming more irritable, perhaps with specific people

- a particular idea keeps entering a person's thoughts

- fear of going mad

- poor appetite

- low mood

- sleep problems

- certain objects or people seem to assume a special significance or meaning

- thoughts racing

- laughing out loud for no apparent reason.

6 Identify three forms of early intervention which may prevent full relapse.

In identifying early interventions you may have focused upon adjustment of medication and/or other actions such as crisis counselling, identifying and managing particular stressors, and general assistance and support to the individual and family. All of these interventions may have merit in staving off a full relapse of the individual's mental state.

7 Describe the role of the Case Manager.

The Case Manager is a broker of care. The interests of the clients are represented in order to gain access to the best possible services. Key elements of the role are:

- assessment
- monitoring
- advocacy.

Appendix two

STRUCTURED PSYCHOEDUCATION PROGRAMME: AN EXAMPLE

Session one

The aims of this session are to introduce the programme to relatives in detail, to discuss the needs of relatives in relation to both professional services and the sufferer, and to raise awareness about schizophrenia from a sufferer's and relatives' perspectives.

1 Introductions to group participants.

2 Outline of four-session programme and format.

3 Discussion – the needs of families and friends when not kept informed, the professional response and current research into schizophrenia, and network support.

4 Video – brief clip from tape which deals with the question 'what is schizophrenia?'.

5 Discussion – what is schizophrenia? Brainstorm what it means to group participants.

6 Summary.

7 Assignment.

Each group participant to read booklets dealing with the issues of 'what is schizophrenia?' and 'help with schizophrenia'.

Session two

The main aims of this session are to focus on the causes of schizophrenia that the relatives/friends are familiar with, and to introduce the stress-vulnerability model of schizophrenia.

1 Review assignment.

2 Audio tape and discussion – listen to the audio tape (dealing with the impact of schizophrenia on relatives and friends, stigma, confusion, worries about guilt/causes, grief and loss).

3 Discussion – what are the relatives' perceptions of the causes of schizophrenia?

4 Introduce the concept of the stress-vulnerability model of schizophrenia, based on what is known about causes.

5 Assignment – relatives to find out the symptoms their family member is currently experiencing, or used to experience. Also the names and contact numbers of their family member's care team.

Session three

The main aims of this session are to discuss in detail the symptoms of schizophrenia that relatives are familiar with, to introduce the concept of positive and negative symptoms and to begin to understand coping strategies.

1 Review assignment.

2 Video 'Understanding Schizophrenia'. Brainstorm the symptoms relatives are familiar with (positive and negative). Introduce the concept of positive and negative symptoms. What control do patients have over their experiences? What makes symptoms easier or harder to cope with?

3 Discussion – of the past problems relating to their family member's schizophrenia. How did they cope with their family member? What did they say or do to handle those situations?

Session four

The main aim of this session is to discuss coping and handling situations that arise from having a relative/friend with schizophrenia.

Discussion – general discussion about coping with symptoms. What makes them worse? What makes them better?

Key facts:

- It's natural to feel angry and frustrated when somebody in the home is suffering from symptoms.

- Stress within the household should be kept to a minimum (hostility, criticism, over-involvement).

- It's important that you take care of yourself and continue to live a full life.

- When problems arise it helps to solve them together in a structured way.

- It is important to know where to go for help and to be aware of what services exist *before* you need them.

- Try to maintain contact with friends, relatives and colleagues.

- Specific strategies for specific symptoms can be adopted following assessment of problems. Help with this can be sought from the primary nurse, the care team or rehab staff.

- Remember that the problem behaviours are caused by schizophrenia and not by the individual.

Appendix three

DEVELOPMENT ISSUES FOR PRIMARY CARE TEAMS

To increase effectiveness, primary care teams may need to carry out the following:

- **Identification of local/city-wide/national mental health resources for information and advice: producing a mental health resource directory.**

  Community mental health teams should produce a mental health resource directory that will be located in each GP practice for use by the primary care team (both professional and administration and clerical staff). This would assist the team by directing people with less severe mental health problems towards appropriate community support, helping to prioritise interventions and reduce the amount of inappropriate referrals to the community mental health team over time.

- **Identification of support agencies the primary care team can access at a local level, e.g.:**

  - housing offices

  - counselling services

  - social services support/specialist mental health

  - psychotherapy

  - drug/alcohol services

  - women's/men's support groups.

  This should include clear local information and description of the service; who can access them and how; full address, telephone numbers, contact person, bus route, etc. (this will facilitate access, thereby reducing potential distress).

- **Assessment of training need of the primary care teams in relation to mental health issues/developments.**

  It is essential to obtain a good level of knowledge and expertise in each practice and to target mental health education and information based on the overall needs of the PCT.

- **Development of mental health training programmes for the primary care teams.**

  This would be based on the assessment of training need and include all team members, including reception and administration staff. It is essential to use the skills and expertise of the primary care team in the delivery of any agreed training programme to reduce time and pressure on the mental health team.

- **Mental illness needs assessment to assist in SMI focus and development of priority systems.**

  This may be undertaken by the Public Health Consultant. It is useful to examine the psychiatric morbidity in the defined geographical area, giving a baseline from which the mental health team can describe their current and future work.

- **Development of SMI practice registers in practice**.

This would include:

- socio-demographic data

- clinical data

- service contacts

- practice policy recall (Strathdee, 1992).

The case registers held within each practice are essential to the maintenance of a SMI focus, ensuring that those who are in contact with secondary care are supported by the workings of the CPA, while identifying those who are provided for in primary care settings.

- **CPA developments in primary care.**

This would include the following:

- how the CPA works

- how the CPA benefits the GP/primary care team

- who should be on the CPA in the practice.

- **Support developments at practice level in the management of people with minor mental health problems, e.g. with:**

- anxiety and depression

- postnatal depression

- assessment and prioritising.

- **Development of systems of casework support to PCT members.**

Develop systems of casework support from the CMHT and CMHN to district nurses, practice nurses, health visitors and school nurses, with a view to preventing referral on to mental health services. This would also involve a focus upon promotion of positive mental health, reducing inappropriate labelling and the stigma of referral to the mental health team.

- **Provide CMHT assessment/screening clinics at individual practice level.**

These clinics would assist in shared care and collaborative working practice, improving communication between primary and secondary care, altering referral patterns to mental health services and reducing the incidence of inappropriate referrals. As such, these clinics would be ideally placed to assist in the early detection of SMI and provide an opportunity to commence early psychosocial interventions for individuals and their families. Assessment and screening clinics can provide the GP with quick access and regular contact with community mental health teams, improving communications and relationships between primary and secondary care services.

- **Development of consultant out-patient clinics in primary care.**

This would improve individual choice for patients, and increase clinic attendance rates by reprovision of services at a local level. There is also the added benefit of reducing myths and stigma of mental illness by bringing issues down to primary care level. Low (1988) reminds us of the further benefits of reduction of hospital admissions, citing a study by Tyrer (1984) where there was an increased referral rate to secondary care of 20% when clinics moved into primary care.

- **Develop recall policies for regular physical health checks for the SMI practice population.**

Practice nurses would be involved in the use of their practice case register of SMI and would ensure all were offered annual physical health screening, contacting the key worker under the CPA if problems arose.

- **Liaison with community drug and alcohol services.**

The emerging agenda of people who present to GPs with mental health problems and use drugs, including problematic alcohol consumption, can make assessment work and treatment more difficult for all involved. It is these issues that can be addressed by the CMHN and CMHT providing invaluable liaison with community drug and alcohol services.

- **Integration to care programming.**

The development of the CPA assists communication between the key worker and primary care team, ensuring follow-up for those who are most in need. It is an integral part of the role of key worker to develop liaison and communication at a primary care level and facilitate teams working together. People suffering a range of mental health problems will be known to practitioners in primary care and may have involvement from other team members. It is important for agreement between each practice and mental health team members to be established around mental health developments, and that clear boundaries and protocols are set in relation to who is the priority group and how other presenting mental health problems are dealt with.

OBJECTIVES FOR SHARED CARE/COLLABORATIVE WORKING (TURNER, 1996)

- Improve services to patients'/clients' carers and families.
- Reduction of stigma for people with mental health problems.
- Reduction of cost for GPs referring on to secondary care services.
- Increased communication between PCT and secondary specialist mental health and social services.
- More appropriate use of existing community services.
- More appropriate use of health and social service resources.
- Development of best practice mental health protocols in primary care.
- Provision of education and support to patients, carers and families.
- Provision of mental health education and promotion.

These service objectives are supported by the development of resource materials. The Department of Health NHS Executive commissioned a series of projects that have resulted in the production of *The Primary Mental Health Care Toolkit* (Armstrong, 1997).

The *Toolkit* aims are as follows:

- to provide easy to use (photocopiable) examples to enable primary care teams to develop systematic approaches to the management of common mental health problems

- to suggest referral criteria

- to indicate points at which local arrangements for care may need to be jointly agreed between GPs and secondary care providers

- to provide a framework within which practice nurses can develop their expertise, including a method of identifying people at risk

- to encourage practice teams to improve their knowledge of and work with local agencies, including the voluntary sector.

The *Toolkit* is not intended to be set in stone but is to be used flexibly as a resource for primary care teams to adapt to meet needs at a local level. With this as a basis to develop mental health working practice in primary care, community mental health teams could assist the process by primary care outreach offering support, advice and practical help, with the overall goal of providing a skilled, locally-based service for screening and managing mental health morbidity in their area.

Appendix four

Training practitioners in the use of psychosocial interventions

Despite the often dramatic results of the research into psychosocial interventions, the early intervention studies were criticised on a number of points. The research usually reported upon the clinical input of very experienced and skilled senior practitioners such as Ian Falloon, Nick Tarrier and Christine Barrowclough. On this point it could be argued that perhaps the delivery of psychosocial interventions might be beyond the realms of competence of ordinary practitioners, or it was merely the exposure to 'expert' attention which accounted for the improvements in outcomes. Moreover, the clinical work itself has often only continued for the length of the particular research project, so that service users or their families only had the chance to engage with the systematic delivery of packages of psychosocial interventions for the duration of the research evaluation. After this time services often reverted back to standard practice. These two criticisms suggested a possible question mark over the extent to which psychosocial interventions could be implemented to make a wholesale impact at the level of service delivery.

Noting this, Brooker and colleagues decided to investigate whether Community Psychiatric Nurses (CPNs) could be taught to deliver psychosocial interventions (Brooker and Butterworth, 1993; Brooker et al., 1994). In doing so they hoped to address the criticisms of the previous research because, if community nurses could be trained to be effective practitioners of psychosocial interventions, then it would demonstrate that the relevant competencies were indeed within the compass of people other than high-profile clinicians. More importantly, positive results would open up the opportunity to train large numbers of community-based staff, CPNs being the most numerous group, in an attempt to address the extent to which psychosocial interventions become incorporated into standard practice and systematised into services. The findings indicated that, even with relatively short training programmes, CPNs could achieve similar results to the original family intervention studies.

The idea of training nurses in these skills, taken together with the realisation that people with a severe mental illness were often neglected by established community services, led to the establishment of the **Thorn Initiative** (Gamble, 1995).

'Thorn' training

The Thorn Nurse Training Initiative was founded with a grant from the Sir Jules Thorn Charitable Trust. It was originally conceived that as such training expanded, 'Thorn' nurses working with the severely mentally ill would become analogous to Macmillan nurses working in cancer care. Although initially offered solely to community mental health nurses, the course and others like it are now open to a range of multidisciplinary practitioners.

The course has three major strands: case management, family interventions and the psychological management of symptoms. The case management teaching covers a variety of different models of organising and coordinating services (see Huxley, 1991). The family management work involves two students co-working with a family in an attempt to address important issues in the family environment. The psychological management module includes training in specific techniques for use with patients experiencing positive and negative symptoms. The students are taught to practise such skills within a problem-centred approach, based upon sound and reliably administered assessments.

There is an emphasis on skills acquisition, with each student carrying a small caseload with whom the clinical work is practised. Because of the priority given to practising skills, there ought to be a direct impact upon patient care in the workplaces of the participating nurses. The demonstrable lack of such a positive consequence is a feature often associated with other practitioner training or continuing education, giving rise to a much commented upon 'theory–practice gap' (Warmuth, 1987; Barriball *et al.*, 1992). The Thorn course itself has been subject to research evaluation of both patient and student outcomes, and the early published results continue to demonstrate the effectiveness of psychosocial interventions and this form of training (Lancashire *et al.*, 1995).

Appendix five

SUMMATIVE ASSESSMENT

In Chapter 4 you were invited to review your understanding of the material within this book by considering PSI in relation to your own practice.

We have included a written assessment which provides an opportunity for you to demonstrate your grasp of the concept of PSI and the principles of interventions within practice. Please complete the following assessment. If you wish to apply for academic credit of level 2 achievement (diploma level) then you can submit this assessment as evidence of achievement. We have not included space in the book for your response to the summative assessment exercise as you may prefer to write on separate paper, with a view to submitting the assessment to a study centre for marking at a later date.

The finished assessment should, if completed well, enable you to claim up to 12 CATs points at a learning institution within higher education. This credit can then count towards achieving a diploma in higher education (you will require 120 level 2 credits in total), which is two-thirds of a degree.

Good luck with your studies!

 Part one

You are the practice nurse for Robert, the patient described in Activity 2.14. Since the time of his last admission you have been in regular contact with Robert and his family and have the facility to liaise if necessary with his CMHT. One of the achievements of your joint working has been engaging the family in addressing the issue of relapse prevention. This has resulted in a strategy of looking out for prodromal (early warning) signs – a list of these is contained in Robert's practice notes.

This day, Robert's father visits the practice and reports that Robert is becoming increasingly suspicious and withdrawn. Both of these are listed as prodromal signs and the family are worried, but are finding it difficult to contact Robert's CPN directly. They have talked to Robert about him coming to see either the GP or his psychiatric consultant, but he refuses. If they press him he becomes sullen and aggressive, which is quite unusual for Robert. The family feel that Robert is depressed, and fear that he may harm himself. In the past he survived a serious suicide attempt.

1 Describe in detail your earlier work with the family, since his last admission.

2 State in detail what actions you should take as a consequence of speaking to Robert's father.

For both answers try to offer a rationale for your actions. Also, pay particular attention to issues around the division of labour between the PCT and the CMHT.

Write your answers on a separate piece of paper.

Part two

Examination of SMI in your practice population. The task is to develop an SMI case register.

You must gather and organise relevant information on those people in your practice with an SMI diagnosis. It should be presented in a manageable form which is useful for your practice.

1 You will need to pay attention to numbers of people with a diagnosis of:

- schizophrenia
- bipolar disorder (manic depression)
- enduring depression (lasting over one year).

2 Structure your information into:

- age ranges
- gender
- contacts with secondary services
- those subject to CPA
- those at risk of:
  - relapse
  - self-harm
  - harm to others
  - self-neglect
  - also having problems with substance use.

3 Outline the benefits you would expect in carrying out this work in your practice for:

- the PCT
- clients and their carers.

References and
further reading

Anderson C, Hogarty G and Reiss D (1980) Family treatment of adult schizophrenic patients: a psychoeducational approach. *Schizophrenia Bulletin.* **6**: 490–505.

Anthony W (1993) Recovery from mental illness: the guiding vision of the mental health service system in the 1990s. *Psychosocial Rehabilitation Journal.* **16**: 11–23.

Anthony W, Cohen M and Cohen B (1983) Philosophy, treatment process, and principles of the psychiatric rehabilitation approach. *New Directions in Mental Health.* **17**: 67–79.

American Psychiatric Association (1980) *Diagnostic and Statistical Manual of Mental Disorders – III.* APA, Washington, DC.

Armstrong E (1997) *The Primary Mental Health Care Toolkit.* Royal College of General Practitioners Unit for Mental Health Education in Primary Care and Institute of Psychiatry Section of Epidemiology and General Practice, supported by the Department of Health, London.

Ayllon T and Azrin N (1968) *The Token Economy.* Appleton-Century-Crofts, New York.

Barker P (1993) Major mental health problems. In H Wright and M Giddley (eds) *Mental Health Nursing: from first principles to practice.* Chapman and Hall, London.

Barriball K, While A and Norman I (1992) Continuing professional education for qualified nurses: a review of the literature. *Journal of Advanced Nursing.* **17**: 1129–40.

Barrowclough C and Tarrier N (1984) Psychosocial interventions with families and their effects on the course of schizophrenia: a review. *Psychological Medicine.* **14**: 629–42.

Barrowclough C, Tarrier N, Watts S *et al.* (1987) Assessing the functional value of relatives' knowledge about schizophrenia: a preliminary report. *British Journal of Psychiatry.* **151**: 1–8.

Barrowclough C and Tarrier N (1992) *Families of Schizophrenic Patients: cognitive-behavioural intervention.* Chapman and Hall, London.

Bazire S (1998) *GP Psychotropic Handbook.* Quay Books, Salisbury.

Beck A, Rush A, Shaw B and Emery G (1979) *Cognitive Therapy of Depression.* Guildford Press, New York.

Bentall R (ed) (1990) *Reconstructing Schizophrenia.* Routledge, London.

Bentall R, Haddock G and Slade P (1994) Cognitive-behavior therapy for persistent auditory hallucinations: from theory to therapy. *Behavior Therapy.* **25**: 51–66.

Bentall R (1996) From cognitive studies of psychosis to cognitive behavioural therapy for psychotic symptoms. In G Haddock and P Slade (eds) *Cognitive Behavioural Interventions with Psychotic Disorders.* Routledge, London.

Berkowitz R (1984) Therapeutic intervention with schizophrenic patients and their families: a description of a clinical research project. *Journal of Family Therapy.* **6**: 211–33.

Birchwood M, Smith J and MacMillan F (1989) Predicting relapse in schizophrenia: the development and implementation of an early signs monitoring system using patients and families as observers, a preliminary investigation. *Psychological Medicine*. **19**: 649–56.

Birchwood M, Smith J, Cochrane R *et al.* (1990) The Social Functioning Scale: the development and validation of a scale of social adjustment for use in family intervention programmes with schizophrenia patients. *British Journal of Psychiatry*. **157**: 853–9.

Birchwood M and Smith J (1991) *Understanding Schizophrenia* (booklet series). Bromsgrove and Redditch Health Authority.

Birchwood M, Macmillan J and Smith J (1992) Early intervention. In M Birchwood and N Tarrier (eds) *Innovations in the Psychological Management of Schizophrenia*. Wiley, Chichester.

Birchwood M and Shepherd G (1992) Controversies and growing points in cognitive-behavioural interventions for people with schizophrenia. *Behavioural Psychotherapy*. **20**: 305–42.

Birchwood M and Tarrier N (eds) (1992) *Innovations in the Psychological Management of Schizophrenia*. Wiley, Chichester.

Bollini P, Pampallona S, Orza M *et al.* (1994) Antipsychotic drugs: is more worse? A meta-analysis of published randomized controlled trials. *Psychological Medicine*. **24**: 307–16.

Brooker C (1990*a*) The health education needs of families caring for a schizophrenic relative and the potential role for community psychiatric nurses. *Journal of Advanced Nursing*. **15**: 1092–8.

Brooker C (1990*b*) Expressed emotion and psychosocial intervention: a review. *International Journal of Nursing Studies*. **27**: 267–76.

Brooker C and Butterworth T (1991) Working with families caring for a relative with schizophrenia: the evolving role of the community psychiatric nurse. *International Journal of Nursing Studies*. **28**: 189–200.

Brooker C, Barrowclough C and Tarrier N (1992) Evaluating the impact of training community psychiatric nurses to educate relatives about schizophrenia. *Journal of Clinical Nursing*. **1**: 19–25.

Brooker C and Butterworth T (1993) Training in psychosocial intervention: the impact on the role of community psychiatric nurses. *Journal of Advanced Nursing*. **18**: 583–90.

Brooker C, Falloon I, Butterworth A *et al.* (1994) The outcome of training community psychiatric nurses to deliver psychosocial intervention. *British Journal of Psychiatry*. **165**: 222–30.

Brown G, Carstairs G and Topping G (1958) The post-hospital adjustment of chronic mental patients. *Lancet*. **ii**: 685–9.

Brown G, Monck E, Carstairs G and Wing J (1962) Influence of family life on the course of schizophrenia disorders. *British Journal of Preventative and Social Medicine*. **16**: 55–68.

Brown G, Birley J and Wing J (1972) Influence of family life on the course of schizophrenia disorders: replication. *British Journal of Psychiatry*. **121**: 241–58.

Brown W and Herz L (1989) Response to neuroleptic drugs as a device for classifying schizophrenia. *Schizophrenia Bulletin.* **15**: 123–8.

Caplan G (1974) The family as a support system. In G Caplan and M Killilea (eds) *Support Systems and Mutual Help: multidisciplinary explorations*, pp. 19–36. Grune and Stratton, New York.

Carlsson A and Lindqvuist M (1963) Effect of chlorpromazine or haloperidol on formation of 3-methoxytyramine and normetanephrine in mouse brain. *Acta Pharmacologica et Toxicologica.* **20**: 140–4.

Chadwick P and Lowe C (1990) The measurement and modification of delusional beliefs. *Journal of Consulting and Clinical Psychology.* **58**: 225–32.

Clinical Standards Advisory Group Committee on Schizophrenia (1995) *Schizophrenia. Volume 1. Report of a CSAG Committee on Schizophrenia.* HMSO, London.

Cohen S and Wills T (1985) Stress, social support and the buffering hypothesis. *Psychological Bulletin.* **98**: 310–57.

Day J, Wood G, Dewey M and Bentall R (1995) A self-rating scale for measuring neuroleptic side effects: validation in a group of schizophrenic patients. *British Journal of Psychiatry.* **166**: 650–3.

Delay J, Deniker P and Harl J (1952) Utilisation en therapeutique psychiatrique d'une phenothiazine d'action centrale elective. *Annales Medico-Psychologiques.* **2**: 112–17.

Department of Health (1993) *The Health of the Nation: Key Area Handbook: Mental Illness.* HMSO, London.

Department of Health (1995) *Building Bridges: a guide to arrangements for inter-agency working for the care and protection of severely mentally ill people.* HMSO, London.

Department of Health (1996a) *Primary Care: the future – choice and opportunity.* HMSO, London.

Department of Health (1998a) *Our Healthier Nation. A contract for health.* The Stationery Office, London.

Department of Health (1998b) National Service Frameworks. Health Service Circular HSC 1998/074. NHS Executive, London.

Doane J, Goldstein M, Miklowitz D and Falloon I (1986) The impact of individual and family treatment on the affective climate of families of schizophrenics. *British Journal of Psychiatry.* **148**: 279–87.

Falloon I (1986) Family stress and schizophrenia. *Psychiatric Clinics of North America.* **9**: 165–81.

Falloon I (1992) Early intervention for first episodes of schizophrenia: a preliminary study. *Psychiatry.* **55**: 4–14.

Falloon I, Boyd J and McGill C (1984) *Family Care of Schizophrenia.* Guildford Press, New York.

Falloon I, Boyd J, McGill C *et al.* (1985) Family management in the prevention of morbidity of schizophrenia. *Archives of General Psychiatry.* **42**: 887–96.

Falloon I, Krekorian H, Shanahan W, Laporta M and McLees S (1990) The Buckingham Project: a comprehensive mental health service based upon behavioural psychotherapy. *Behaviour Change.* **7**(2): 51–7.

Falloon I, Laporta L, Fadden G and Graham-Hole V (1993) *Managing Stress in Families.* Routledge, London.

Flannery D and Link I (1986) A model comprehensive family programme for relatives of adult schizophrenics. *Psychosocial Rehabilitation Journal.* **9**: 15–24.

Gallagher A, Dinan T and Baker L (1994) The effects of varying auditory input on schizophrenic hallucinations: a replication. *British Journal of Medical Psychology.* **67**: 67–76.

Gamble C (1995) The Thorn Nurse Training Initiative. *Nursing Standard.* **9**(15): 31–4.

Gilbert P, Harris M, McAdams L and Jeste D (1995) Neuroleptic withdrawal in schizophrenic patients. *Archives of General Psychiatry.* **52**: 173–212.

Goldberg J and Triano-Antidormi L (1992) *Cognitive Rehabilitation.* Hamilton Programme for Schizophrenia, Hamilton, Ontario.

Goldstein M, Rodnick E, Evans J, May P and Steinberg M (1978) Drug and family therapy in the aftercare of acute schizophrenics. *Archives of General Psychiatry.* **35**: 1169–77.

Gournay K (1994) Redirecting the emphasis to serious mental illness. *Nursing Times.* **90**(25): 40–1.

Gournay K and Brooking J (1994) Community nurses in primary health care. *British Journal of Psychiatry.* **165**: 231–8.

Greenberg L, Fine S, Cohen C *et al.* (1988) An interdisciplinary psychoeducation programme for schizophrenic patients and their families in an acute care setting. *Hospital and Community Psychiatry.* **39**: 277–82.

Greenblatt M, Beccara R and Serafetinides E (1982) Social networks and mental health: an overview. *American Journal of Psychiatry.* **139**: 977–84.

Greene R (1978) Auditory hallucination reduction: first person singular therapy. *Journal of Contemporary Psychotherapy.* **9**: 167–70.

Haddock G and Slade P (eds) (1996) *Cognitive-Behavioural Interventions with Psychotic Disorders.* Routledge, London.

Hallam A (1997) Through a glass darkly: media images of mental illness. *Mental Health Research Review.* **4**: 10–11.

Hansen D, St Lawrence J and Christoff K (1985) Effects of interpersonal problem-solving training with chronic aftercare patients on problem-solving component skills and effectiveness of solutions. *Journal of Consulting and Clinical Psychology.* **53**: 167–74.

Hatfield A (1990) *Family Education in Mental Illness.* Guildford Press, New York.

Hertz M and Melville C (1980) Relapse in schizophrenia. *American Journal of Psychiatry.* **137**: 801–12.

Hirsch S (1986) Clinical treatment of schizophrenia. In P Bradley and S Hirsch (eds) *The Psychopharmocology and Treatment of Schizophrenia.* Oxford University Press, Oxford.

Hogarty G, Anderson C, Reiss D *et al.* (1986) Family psychoeducation, social skills training and maintenance chemotherapy in the aftercare treatment of schizophrenia. *Archives of General Psychiatry.* **43**: 633–42.

Hubbard J, Midha K, Hawes E *et al.* (1993) Metabolism of phenothiazine and butyrophenone antipsychotic drugs: a review of some recent research findings and clinical implications. *British Journal of Psychiatry.* **163**(25): 22–31.

Huxley P (1991) Effective case management for mentally ill people: the relevance of recent evidence from the USA for case management services in the United Kingdom. *Social Work and Social Sciences Review.* **2**(3): 192–203.

Huxley P (1993) Case management and care management in community care. *British Journal of Social Work.* **23**: 365–81.

James D (1983) The experimental treatment of two cases of auditory hallucinations. *British Journal of Psychiatry.* **143**: 515–16.

Jenkins R (1992) Developments in the primary care of mental illness: a forward look. *International Review of Psychiatry.* **4**: 237–42.

Johnson C, Gilmore J and Shenoy R (1983) Thought-stopping and anger induction in the treatment of hallucinations and obsessional ruminations. *Psychotherapy: Theory, Research, Practice.* **20**: 445–8.

Johnstone L (1993) Family management of 'schizophrenia': its assumptions and contradictions. *Journal of Mental Health.* **2**: 255–69.

Kane J and Marder S (1993) Psychopharmacologic treatment of schizophrenia. *Schizophrenia Bulletin.* **19**: 287–302.

King M (1992) Management of patients with schizophrenia in general practice. *British Journal of General Practice.* **42**: 310–11.

Kingdon D and Turkington D (1991) Preliminary report: the use of cognitive-behaviour therapy and a normalizing rationale in schizophrenia. *Journal of Nervous and Mental Disease.* **179**: 207–11.

Kingdon D, Turkington D and John C (1994) Cognitive-behaviour therapy of schizophrenia: the amenability of delusions and hallucinations to reasoning. *British Journal of Psychiatry.* **164**: 581–7.

Kingdon D, Turkington D and Beck AT (1995) *Cognitive-behavior Therapy of Schizophrenia.* Psychology Press.

Krawiecka M, Goldberg D and Vaughan M (1977) A standardised psychiatric assessment scale for rating chronic psychotic patients. *Acta Psychiatrica Scandinavica.* **55**: 299–308.

Kyle S and Taylor P (1983) Developing a group for friends and families of schizophrenics: a hospital model. *Canada's Mental Health.* **3**: 14–25.

Lam D (1991) Psychosocial family intervention in schizophrenia: a review of empirical studies. *Psychological Medicine.* **21**: 423–41.

Lancashire S, Haddock G, Tarrier N *et al.* (1995) The impact of training community psychiatric nurses to use psychosocial interventions with people who have serious mental health problems: the Thorn Nurse Training Project. *International Journal of Psychiatric Nursing Research.* **2**(1): 124–33.

Leff J, Kuipers L, Berkowitz R *et al.* (1982) A controlled trial of social intervention in the families of schizophrenic patients. *British Journal of Psychiatry.* **141**: 121–34.

Liberman R, Teigen J, Patterson R and Baker V (1973) Reducing delusional speech in chronic paranoid schizophrenics. *Journal of Applied Behaviour Analysis.* **6**: 57–64.

Liberman R, Falloon I and Aitchison R (1984) Multiple family therapy for schizophrenia: a behavioural problem-solving approach. *Psychosocial Rehabilitation Journal.* **7**: 60–77.

Lindstrom L and Wieselgren I (1996) Schizophrenia and antipsychotic somatic treatment. *International Journal of Technology Assessment in Health Care.* **12**: 573–84.

Low B (1988) Psychiatric clinics in different settings. A case register study. *British Journal of Psychiatry.* **153**: 243–5.

Margo A, Hemsley D and Slade P (1981) The effects of varying auditory input on schizophrenic hallucinations. *British Journal of Psychiatry.* **139**: 122–7.

McCann G and Clancy B (1996) Family matters. *Nursing Times.* **92**(7): 46–8.

McGill C, Falloon I, Boyd J and Wood-Silverio C (1983) Family educational intervention in the treatment of schizophrenia. *Hospital and Community Psychiatry.* **34**: 934–8.

McKeown M and Clancy B (1995) Media influence on societal perceptions of mental illness. *Mental Health Nursing.* **15**: 10–12.

Mental Health Act Commission and the Sainsbury Centre (1997) *The National Visit.* Sainsbury Centre for Mental Health, London.

Mental Health Nursing Review Team (1994) *Working in Partnership: a collaborative approach to Care. Report of the Mental Health Nursing Review Team* [Butterworth Report]. HMSO, London.

Miller T (1989) Group psychotherapy; a psychoeducative model for schizophrenic patients and their families. *Perspectives in Psychiatric Care.* **25**: 5–9.

Moxley D (1989) *The Practice of Case Management.* Sage, London.

Nelson H, Thrasher S and Barnes T (1991) Practical ways of relieving auditory hallucinations. *British Medical Journal.* **302**: 307.

Nydegger R (1972) The elimination of hallucinatory and delusional behaviour by verbal conditioning and assertive training: a case study. *Journal of Behaviour Therapy and Experimental Psychiatry.* **3**: 225–7.

Onyett S and Cambridge P (1992) *Case Management: issues in practice.* Chapman and Hall, London.

Reid A, Lang C and O'Neil T (1993) Services for schizophrenic patients and their families: what they say they need. *Behavioural Psychotherapy.* **21**: 107–13.

Reybee J and Kinch B (1973) *Treatment of auditory hallucinations using focusing.* Unpublished study.

References and further reading

Romme M and Escher S (1993) *Accepting Voices*. MIND Publications, London.

Rothman J (1991) A model of case management: toward empirically based practice. *Social Work*. **36**: 520–8.

Royal College of Psychiatrists and Royal College of General Practitioners (1993) *Report of a Joint Working Group on Shared Care*. Occasional Paper 60. RCGP, London.

Silverstone T and Turner P (1991) *Drug Treatment in Psychiatry* (4th edn). Routledge, London.

Slade P (1972) The effects of systematic desensitisation on auditory hallucinations. *Behaviour Research and Therapy*. **10**: 85–91.

Slade P (1990) The behavioural and cognitive treatment of psychotic symptoms. In R Bentall (ed) *Reconstructing Schizophrenia*. Routledge, London.

Slade P and Bentall R (1988) *Sensory Deception: a scientific analysis of hallucinations*. Croom Helm, London.

Smith J and Birchwood M (1987) Specific and non-specific effects of educational intervention with families living with a schizophrenic relative. *British Journal of Psychiatry*. **150**: 645–52.

Sohlberg M and Mateer C (1989) *Introduction to Cognitive Rehabilitation: theory and practice*. Guilford Press, New York.

Strathdee G (1992) The interface between psychiatry and primary care in the management of schizophrenic patients in the community. In R Jenkins, V Field and R Young (eds) *The Primary Care of Schizophrenia*. HMSO, London.

Strathdee G, Kendrick T, Cohen A and Thompson K (1996) *A General Practitioner's Guide to Managing Long-Term Mental Health Disorders*. Sainsbury Centre for Mental Health, London.

Tarrier N (1992) Management and modification of residual positive psychotic symptoms. In M Birchwood and N Tarrier (eds) (1992) *Innovations in the Psychological Management of Schizophrenia*. Wiley, Chichester.

Tarrier N and Barrowclough C (1986) Providing information to relatives about schizophrenia: some comments. *British Journal of Psychiatry*. **149**: 458–63.

Tarrier N, Barrowclough C, Vaughan C *et al.* (1988) The community management of schizophrenia. A controlled trial of a behavioural intervention with families to reduce relapse. *British Journal of Psychiatry*. **153**: 532–42.

Tarrier N, Harwood S, Yusupoff L *et al.* (1990) Coping strategy enhancement: a method of treating residual schizophrenic symptoms. *Behavioural Psychotherapy*. **18**: 283–93.

Thornicroft G and Bebbington P (1989) Deinstitutionalisation: from hospital closure to service development. *British Journal of Psychiatry*. **155**: 739–53.

Turner T (1996) Managing schizophrenia in the community: the role of the GP. *Clinician*. **14**: 9–17.

Tyrer P (1984) Psychiatric clinics in general practice: an extension of community care. *British Journal of Psychiatry.* **145**: 9–14.

Vaughan C and Leff J (1976*a*) The influence of family and social factors on the course of psychiatric illness: a comparison of schizophrenic and depressed neurotic patients. *British Journal of Psychiatry.* **129**: 125–37.

Vaughan C and Leff J (1976*b*) The measurement of expressed emotion in the families of psychiatric patients. *British Journal of Social Clinical Psychology.* **15**: 157–65.

Walker A (ed) (1982) *Community Care: the family, the state and social policy.* Blackwell/Martin Robertson, Oxford.

Warmuth J (1987) In search of the impact of continuing education. *Journal of Continuing Education in Nursing.* **18**(1): 4–7.

Watts F, Powell E and Austin S (1973) The modification of abnormal beliefs. *British Journal of Medical Psychology.* **46**: 359–63.

Weil M and Karls J (1985) *Case Management in Human Service Practice.* Jossey-Bass, London.

Wing J, Cooper J and Sartorius N (1974) *The Measurement and Classification of Psychiatric Symptoms.* Cambridge University Press, Cambridge.

Zelitch S (1980) Helping the family cope: workshops for families of schizophrenics. *Health and Social Work.* **5**: 47–52.

Zubin J and Spring B (1977) Vulnerability: a new view of schizophrenia. *Journal of Abnormal Psychology.* **86**: 260–6.